# EATING
# ETHICALLY

—

# JONATHAN K. CRANE

# EATING ETHICALLY

Religion and Science

for a Better Diet

COLUMBIA UNIVERSITY PRESS
NEW YORK

Columbia University Press
*Publishers Since 1893*
New York   Chichester, West Sussex
cup.columbia.edu
Copyright © 2018 Jonathan K. Crane
All rights reserved

Library of Congress Cataloging-in-Publication Data

Names: Crane, Jonathan K. (Jonathan Kadane), author.
Title: Eating ethically : religion and science for a better diet / Jonathan K. Crane.
Description: New York : Columbia University Press, 2018. | Includes
  bibliographical references and index.
Identifiers: LCCN 2017019389 (print) | LCCN 2017046619 (ebook) | ISBN
  9780231545877 (electronic) | ISBN 9780231173445 (cloth : alk. paper)
Subjects: LCSH: Food consumption—Moral and ethical aspects. | Food—Moral
  and ethical aspects. | Food—Religious aspects.
Classification: LCC TX357 (ebook) | LCC TX357 .C68 2018 (print) | DDC
  178—dc23
LC record available at https://lccn.loc.gov/2017019389

∞

Columbia University Press books are printed on permanent
and durable acid-free paper.
Printed in the United States of America

Cover design: Milenda Nan Ok Lee
Cover images: © Shutterstock

*And know indeed that*
*what kind of a person is,*
*is determined at the table,*
*for there his qualities*
*are revealed and made known.*

—Bahya ben Asher ibn Halawa,
*Shulḥan Shel Arba* (Second Gate) (1255–1340)


*The Vulture eats between his meals*
*And that's the reason why*
*He very, very, rarely feels*
*As well as you and I.*
*His eye is dull, his head is bald,*
*His neck is growing thinner.*
*Oh! What a lesson for us all*
*To only eat at dinner.*

—Hilaire Belloc,
*More Beasts for Worse Children* (1897)

# CONTENTS

## PART IV: I EAT THEREFORE I AM TASTEFUL

—

## PART V: CONCLUSION

—

# PREFACE

S everal years ago, I was looking around in the field of bioethics for discussions about eating-related ailments. I was surprised to find that, compared to other bioethical topics such as beginning- and end-of-life interventions, relatively little had been written on this one. This was true in the field of religious ethics, too. Curious about this gap in the conversation, I dug around in the tradition I know best: Judaism. I soon found a few classic resources suggesting that good health stems from eating well. I was not surprised, because that opinion is well known today. What did surprise me, though, was that the eating well these sources envision differed dramatically from the eating strategies I was more familiar with in the contemporary food environment. They inverted eating's orientation. Intrigued, I dug around some more and found that these were not isolated positions: other religious traditions encouraged similar eating strategies. Philosophers throughout history thought these strategies reasonable; and even contemporary physiology and the scientific study of eating corroborate these old ideas.

I pulled together some preliminary thoughts on these topics into an op-ed piece for the *New York Times*, which was published in March 2013 under the title "The Talmud and Other Diet Books."[1] That brief piece caught the eye of Patrick Fitzgerald, the editor at Columbia University Press, who called me with a simple query: Could this very brief column be made into a book? Ever since that initial conversation Patrick has been a stalwart enthusiast for this project, and for this I am extremely grateful.

I soon found myself reading in such fields as food studies, physiology, satiety studies, religious history (of food), philosophy (of food), cultural studies, medicine, and more. I also observed that dramatic shifts in attitudes toward food and practices in eating were occurring in society generally. A veritable explosion of interest in all things food has happened: just think of the incredible growth of food-centered TV shows and channels, documentaries, book-length journalistic investigations, food clubs, community-supported agriculture, sustainable and organic restaurants, and more that have emerged in the past few years.

I offered an undergraduate class at Emory University on the topic; it was overenrolled. Encouraged, the next year I flipped the classroom so that we were in a kitchen: the students were to plan menus, shop for food, and prep, cook, and serve meals based on weekly themes. By turning the academy on its head, we literally ate our subject matter, whether commodity crops or farmers' markets produce, whether from the Supplemental Nutrition Assistance Program (SNAP) or religious consumptive rituals. That class had a waiting list of over fifty students. When I offered that class again the next year, any student at Emory could take it. Nearly 150 students from every school in the university applied for the twenty spots. I was fortunate to collaborate on those courses with incredible colleagues from across the university: Amy Webb Girard, Mindy Goldstein, Peggy Barlett, Laurence Sperling, Sam Sober, Linda Craighead, Jennifer Frediani, Simona Muratore, Craig Hadley, and Peter Thule, among others. Their wisdom has been invaluable to this project.

Interest in this intersection of food and eating-related ethics, religion, and science has been palpable off campus, too. Over the past several years, various communities around North America have asked me to present on these topics. This project has benefited from the insights, questions, and provocations of audiences at St. John's University, University of St. Thomas, Case Western Reserve University, Mercer University, Georgia Institute of Technology, the Judaism, Science and Medicine Group, the American Society of Bioethics and Humanities, the Commission on Social Action of Reform Judaism, the Chicago Board of Rabbis, Religious Action Center, Temple Beth Am of Seattle, Yom Limmud in Houston, and Congregation Shearith Israel in Atlanta.

I emerged from these conversations convinced that this project should not be merely academic. While of course it should be grounded in solid research, I wanted it to reach a larger audience. I have thus written it for keen readers interested in appreciating the intertwining of religion, science, and philosophy in relation to eating and food. Citations are set at the end so the book may be read without distraction; the bibliography suggests further reading. Even as the book makes a cumulative argument, individual chapters are more or less freestanding units. Its many visuals either augment or are integral to the story.

From the book's earliest inception, the faculty, staff, and students at the Center for Ethics at Emory University have been exceptional colleagues, mentors, interlocutors, and, most important, commensal partners. Without them, I could not have developed the ideas or carved out the time to build this project and its related courses.

Closer to home, I am thankful to Dancing Goats, our neighborhood caffeine dispensary, where stimulating conversations were never lacking and where I wrote substantial portions of this book. Through the years I had many fruitful conversations with David Goldstein, Leah Garces and Ben Lopman, Aaron Gross, Janine Franco and Alan Pinstein, Jaci and Jon Effron, Mike and Dana Geller, Lisa and Moses Staimez, Charles and Nola Miller, Barbara and Peter Cohen. My wife, Lindy, and our sons—Nadav, Amitai, and Rafael—are my constant and beloved table partners, always ready for cooking up and enjoying a tasty meal.

This book is dedicated to my parents, Kathryn and Garry Crane, at whose table I grew up. They nourished me with an appreciation for good food made at home from real ingredients, best eaten with loved ones at a table without corners. Because of them, I came to understand that eating well is a daily and lifelong choice.

# EATING
# ETHICALLY

—

# EATING UNWELL

---

*For eating is that indispensable vital activity*
*closest to the mindlessly natural,*
*yet it is also influenced by the emergence*
*of mind and culture.*

—Leon Kass, *The Hungry Soul* (1999)

# 1

# FULL OF OURSELVES

*Eating is a scandal at the heart of human life.*

—Alec Irwin, "Devoured by God" (2001)

T hough it may seem in this era of superabundance that human eating has recently gone haywire, we have always struggled with understanding ourselves as eaters and what constitutes eating well. Evidence of our contemporary malaise flashes in the headlines daily, accosting us with pictures of sagging waists and charts of exploding health-care costs due to food-related maladies. We see it in the shocking disparities between those who have access to a range of decent foods and those who do not. Our purchases of certain foods, like meats and commodity crops, also create significant environmental effects. We have established convoluted legal and economic incentives that perversely and frequently negatively impact farmers and laborers. From failing personal health to faltering biospheric integrity, our current consumptive practices are increasingly proving to be not just unhealthy but altogether maladaptive.

Why? Why has our eating become so troublesome? Why has eating become in so many ways a deadly enterprise? Surely we humans have not always eaten so poorly; we would not have survived as a species were that true. So how can we make contemporary eating more adaptive, healthy, ethical? What might a better diet look like?

Pursuing such questions requires focusing more on eating than on food. Let us consider our assumptions about eating, because how we think about eating necessarily shapes how we eat, what we eat, when, with whom, and why.

Eating is more than a mere physical activity. Yet because we eat so habitually we have become inured to it: rarely do we pause to consider what we are eating and why we are eating this and not that. We hardly stop to think what being an eater implies in the first place.

Instead we are apt to ply ourselves mindlessly with what we believe is food. Many of us do this frequently, often in strange settings, like moving vehicles or dark rooms with flickering screens surrounded by people with whom we do not interact. We order sumptuous meals packed with silent killers. Our companies and schools and retailers cram foodstuffs into stairwell dispensaries and cashier stations to surround us with consumables, lest we go hungry for even a moment. Ironically, our hospitals often outsource cafés to fast-food chains that sell precisely the stuff that sends consumers back to the medical clinics, forging a perversely self-reinforcing and symbiotic relationship that extracts more and more money from the very people the hospitals assist.

We tease ourselves with food constantly. We bombard ourselves with advertisements touting flavors of the week and diets of the month. These ads whet our appetites, but they fade from the mind so quickly that we are soon ready for the next round. Our bodies hardly have time to adapt as we push the tantalizing stuff into ourselves. Sales of prepared food, especially combination or "combo" sales, arrest our attention and lead us to open our wallets. We have come to mistake the convenient and cheap for the nutritious. We favor longevity of our food: just note the manufactured foodstuffs lining the shelves at gas stations. Many are canned or packed with artificial preservatives and strange colors, making them more synthetic than biological; they are designed to allure and endure more than nourish. Nevertheless we pick them up, purchase them, open their wrappers, take a bite, quickly savor, swallow, and move on—hardly thinking about any of this.

Why do we wonder why so many suffer from food-related ills?

To be sure we should pay attention to the food our system produces. We should be concerned how what we consume gets from farm and factory to our grocery stores, restaurants, and bodegas. We should also be wary about the ever-changing diet regimens touted by authorities, as they are frequently influenced by powerful lobbies or vested interests. We should investigate how and why certain populations suffer a severe lack of nutritious foods when other populations enjoy superabundance, because structural injustices and long-standing prejudices are probably at play.

Yet such studies will do little to illuminate what it means to eat and what it means to be an eater. Looking at food distracts us from what we each do with food. No farm, no company, no law, no diet *eats*. In complicated ways, those other entities *feed* us, but we *eat*. So while we must study how our civilization goes about feeding itself, we also need to understand the basic fact that we are eaters: we need to understand what it means *to eat* and *to be eaters*.

## WHAT ABOUT EATING?

Turning our attention to eating itself is a multifaceted task. At one level we need to appreciate the natural biological features of eating. Anatomy, physiology, and the sciences of metabolism, nutrition, and neurobiology of taste intertwine here. These fields focus on the body. At another level, eating necessarily involves other perspectives. For example, I eat foods that come within reach. Because food is what is beyond me, eating is a dynamic relationship between me and that which I consume. It is also a relationship with other eaters. This interactive feature of eating brings in morality, a complicated subject that integrates both philosophical and theological notions of good and bad, right and wrong. Eating "retains its importance and its glory" precisely because of science as well as "its moral history," as the eighteenth-century French gourmand Jean Anthelme Brillat-Savarin observed.[1] It is at once intensely personal and immensely social, both idiosyncratic and universal. Focusing on either its materiality or its socially constructed elements will not suffice; both are integral to understanding eating in all its glory.

What it means to eat and what it means to be eaters has been known for a long time. For example, an ancient author whose work has been canonized in the Bible observed, "There is nothing better for a man than that he should eat and drink. . . . For who eats and who enjoys but myself?"[2] Eating is done by individuals and is something individuals enjoy. Most other endeavors and achievements are like property: they can be passed on to others. Eating, by contrast, is that activity whose benefits redound back to the individual eater, both while the food is being consumed and digested and later, as it nourishes the body.

Many ancient sources speak about eating, about both its benefits and its dangers. While few premodern sources had the scientific insights we have today about the anatomy and physiology of eating, they nevertheless reflected on the material side of eating. I will review those insights in due course in this book. Suffice it to say for now that human musings on eating have been around for millennia and have been robust, scientifically and normatively.

A further question arises, in addition to exploring the nature of eating and what it means to be eaters: What does it means to eat well? Answering this requires, in part, attending to a related issue: What does it mean to eat poorly? There are, of course, many ways to eat poorly. A common concern is when to stop eating. The bigger problem for some, though, is starting to eat in the first place or eating enough. Figuring out when, how, and why to start or stop eating is perhaps no less biologically and ethically fraught than figuring out how to eat well. Indeed, these issues—eating well and starting and stopping eating—are intimately interrelated.

## STUFFED FULL OF PROBLEMS

"I'm stuffed." This short phrase says a great deal. The speaker often means he or she has reached a stage of consumption verging on the uncomfortable (e.g., "I'm so stuffed I can't move!"). Perhaps the speaker has merely attained a level of repletion requiring no more food. Either way, the hosts know they have done their duty, having plied their guests with plentiful food. It is an expression eaters want to say and feeders want to hear, for it means everyone has achieved their respective goals: to be stuffed and to stuff.

This exchange has become so pervasive in our culture, in our restaurants, and at our kitchen tables that it occurs without much notice. Rarely do people pause to consider the phrase's deeper meanings, and they use it after nearly every meal. Some people do pause, however, and would rather avoid likening themselves to the very foods they've eaten, such as stuffed turkey or double-stuffed potatoes, much less to the overly stuffed

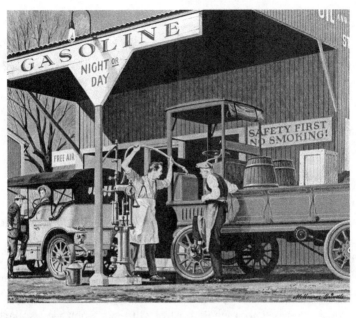

**FIGURE 1.1**

A 1952 Timken-Detroit Axle advertisement.

furniture upon which they so desire to lie down to pant. So instead they push away their plates and say, "I'm full."

What does this mean, to be full? Though "full" has been linked to eating for nearly a thousand years, the expression "I'm full" came into vogue only in the mid-twentieth century, when the automobile was the central figure of American progress and success.[3] For over a century now, we have continued to drive into a gas station, open the gas cap, pour fuel into the tank, and when we resume our journeys the gauge points away from the "E" to the "F." With gas tanks full, our automobiles can go just about anywhere our dreams imagine. With tanks full, they are effective and efficient machines, ideal vehicles onto which we can hitch our aspirations, especially our economic ones. It is unsurprising, then, that the notion of fullness came to be linked with effectiveness and efficiency in the American landscape. This linkage seeped into our own desires to be effective and efficient machines of the burgeoning post–World War II American

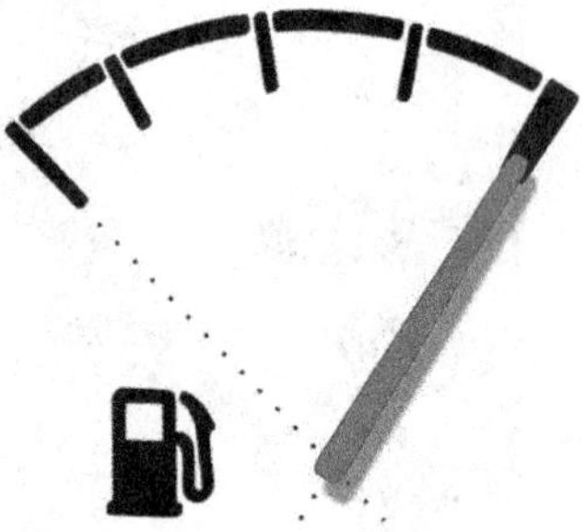

**FIGURE 1.2**

Only a full tank can get you there.

economy. Speaking of ourselves as full at meals became a simple rhetorical strategy to import and superimpose this mechanistic ideal onto our organic selves. When we are full, we are the best of all machines.

Yet this analogy has begun to sputter and stall. Vehicles run well when full, but do stomachs? Do we not suffer indigestion when full, especially when "full to the brim"? Though we fill our gas tanks frequently, do we not expose ourselves to a whole host of ailments when we regularly fill ourselves, particularly when we fill ourselves with questionable foodstuffs that are more akin to toxins than real food? Philosophically, what does it mean to compare ourselves to vehicles? Are we machines that break down and rust? Might there be something insidious in thinking this way, not to mention eating this way? The French philosopher Emmanuel Levinas (1906–1995) thinks so. He argues that privileging fullness is dangerous: it assumes that anything less than being full is less than ideal.[4]

We have come to think that being full is the marker of satisfaction, that being full should be our aim since fullness is life's purpose. Add this philosophical attitude toward fullness to the mechanistic and economic incentive model of fullness, and it is no wonder that fullness became the standard for our eating.

Yet something strange happens when we eat our fill: we become mollified; that is, we become contented with ourselves. Our hunger, our very neediness dissipates. By reestablishing our natural plenitude, we do not need anything else; indeed, we need nothing at all. We lack nothing and we need nothing. All things beyond us are unnecessary and undesirable. As all other things fade into oblivion our metaphysical and physical worlds merge.

In short, when we are full we become full of ourselves. This allows egoism, narcissism, and many other venalities to spawn.

Conversely, according to this worldview, those patterns of eating that do not produce fullness are both metaphysically and physically unsatisfactory. Were I to eat too much or too little and/or inappropriately so that fullness is not achieved, my body would not be satisfied. My fleshy needs would go unmet. When physically unsatisfied I remain needy. To the extent that I am needy, I cannot be my best, true, authentic self. Whether I am hungry, stuffed, or malnourished, I am not fully real: I am unreal. Of course, hunger and malnutrition are real and need careful attention.

This worldview fixated upon fullness assumes the very existence of need as deleterious and undesirable. Need is something to be avoided. Ideal existence has no needs; it is replete and full.

This approach fails life. For life—biological existence itself—is necessarily needy. No biological creature lives only for itself. None is so full of itself that it has no needs. All biological creatures exert energy and in so doing deplete their own stores of energy. In and through living, each creature necessarily becomes needy: its needs to replenish its energy necessarily and constantly reassert themselves. The only way a creature can live is to meet those biological needs constantly, and this is done in part by consuming the world around it. I will say more on this later. For now, though, we should appreciate the fact that any entity that does not need to eat or that has no need to meet, is not a living being.[5] Life is, by definition, needy. Need is therefore not a marker of an insufficiency of being but the marker of the very being of being. Need signifies life. Fullness, by contrast, suggests unlife; fullness—that which is perfectly content—is death.

Eating until one is stuffed or full is obviously problematic. Thinking that eating should produce repletion is similarly troublesome. We need a change in both our eating habits and the ways we speak and think about eating. But a change to what?

We could, for example, invoke the common Japanese phrase *Gochiso sama deshita*, which means "That was quite a feast." This would orient our attention away from ourselves and toward the quality and quantity of the food provided in a meal. Yet how healthy is it to feast at every meal? And if we are not feasting at a meal, what exactly are we doing? Or we could use the Hindi word *bas*, which means "enough," "plenty," or "stop" and is often said while gesturing to cover one's plate. It could mean that one has enough food on one's plate and a server or host should not add more. It could also mean that one is busy eating and should be left alone while continuing to stuff oneself.

Certainly these and other phrases from cultures around the world could enrich the ways we think and speak about eating. Yet they also have their own limitations and quirks. These two examples, for instance, urge us to pay attention to the bounty of a meal just completed or what is on our plate right now. That is, they turn our attention to cues external to our own bodies. No doubt many things beyond our bodies influence our eating: the physical setting of an eating event, the quantity and quality of the food, the social environment, and more. Appreciating how such external forces influence eating is surely called for.

Yet where is the eater? Where am I, the one who eats, when I invoke such phrases or take on such perspectives? Lest we risk harming or forgetting ourselves, we need a way of speaking and thinking about eating that reflects and honors the fact that we are indeed eaters.

## INTO THE UNKNOWN

One of the earliest Nobel Prizes in Medicine was awarded to the nineteenth-century Russian physiologist Ivan Pavlov. Now famous for his work on reflexes and dogs, he was given this extraordinary award in 1904 for his groundbreaking studies on the physiology of digestion. By creating fistulas (open holes) along the digestive tract, he was able to observe the digestive organs as they functioned within living organisms. Before his innovative technique, any analysis of their interactions with the larger organism had to be derived from extracted—that is, dead—organs. Pavlov's revolutionary technique opened up the internal workings of the body so that living tissues continued to interact even as they were being observed and tested. The living body, not dead pieces cut from it, now became the source for medical knowledge, an advancement that radically changed medicine's powers.

Pavlov's fascination with the digestive tract was purposive. For him, it was the basis of all life. As he said in his Nobel Prize acceptance speech:

It is not accidental that all phenomena of human life are dominated by the search for daily bread—the oldest link connecting all living things, man included, with the surrounding nature. Food finding its way into the organism where it undergoes certain changes—is decomposed, enters into new combinations and again dissociates—represents the process of life in all its fullness, from such elementary physical properties of the organism as weight, inertia, etc., all the way to the highest manifestations of human nature. Precise knowledge of what happens to the food entering the organism must be the subject of ideal physiology, the physiology of the future. Present-day physiology can but engage in the continuous accumulation of material for the achievement of this distant aim.[6]

Pavlov's statement is significant: life relies upon eating and food. Appreciating and perhaps improving "all phenomena of human life" thus require appreciating the fact that eating is more than just a regular activity. Eating is that activity upon which all other human endeavors depend.

However basic or foundational eating may be, comprehending its myriad intricacies and interactions remains a challenge. What Pavlov said in 1904 about the physiology of eating—that precise knowledge of digestion is the subject of physiology of the future—may be reiterated today. Though it is indisputable that in the past century science has dramatically increased our collective knowledge of how digestion occurs and its powerful impact on our overall health, the contemporary science of digestion has not yet achieved perfect comprehension of the inner workings of the gut. Neurobiology, sociobiology, psychology, and psychiatry, not to mention anatomy, physiology, and chemistry, are still making huge strides alongside nutrition science, environmental science, dietetics, and many other fields; they all continue to ever improve our collective understanding of eating and food. Still, perfect knowledge eludes.

Perhaps such perfect knowledge will forever evade our grasp. The great nineteenth-century German philosopher Friedrich Nietzsche once wondered, "What is known of the moral effects of different foods? Is there any philosophy of nutrition?"[7] Even if all philosophers, scientists, and everyone else, for that matter, engaged in a collective effort to answer such questions, they would be unable to exhaust the topic. To support his point, Nietzsche parenthetically observed, "The incessantly erupting clamour for and against vegetarianism proves that there is still no such philosophy!"[8] Even a century and a half later the debate on vegetarianism continues to rage. Indeed, the cacophony of claims and counterclaims about this diet or that one speaks to the truth Nietzsche identifies.

While scientists cannot develop perfect data on eating, and philosophers cannot calm their squabbles, eating remains a great unknown. Though eating is an enduring mystery, we must continuously wonder about it: our very lives depend upon it. Eating's hidden features and dynamics manifest a profound impact upon our well-being and on our very notions of being. Who we are is caught up in our eating. Even though we may never attain perfect knowledge of either the physical or philosophical layers of eating, our very existence depends on pursuing such knowledge. In brief, while eating may remain incomprehensible in toto, we ignore it at our peril.

## INTO THE KNOWN

A place to begin is with ourselves. We take inspiration from the Greek imperative "Know thyself" (*Gnŏthi seauton*), etched in stone at the Temple of Apollo at Delphi. A first step to knowing ourselves as eaters is to acknowledge that heretofore we have, for the most part, poorly understood ourselves as such and that our eating practices frequently reflect this sad truism. In part because we know too little about ourselves as eaters, many of us eat so poorly that we are eating ourselves if not to death then at least to ill health. How can we better know ourselves as eaters? What ideas might enable us to eat better and thereby nourish ourselves well?

To answer these and associated questions, I draw from a diverse range of sources of wisdom and knowledge, specifically religion, philosophy, and physiology. These three may seem an odd set of resources since these disciplines rarely address or respect one another, yet each adds unique insights about the what and the why of eating. They complement one another, often filling the others' lacunae. Where one may expand upon how eating occurs, another can address for what ends eating happens. While one teaches why eating is to be valued a particular way, another situates eating and its objects in a larger dynamic field of relationships. Eating is so multidimensional that no single perspective or academic discipline can adequately exhaust the subject matter. Indeed, eating is a necessarily physiological phenomenon no less than it is a heady enterprise and theological conundrum. Appreciating this fact about eating is best done by integrating and intertwining the resources these disciplines offer.

I begin, in chapter 2, by asking: What is poor eating? It could be said there are as many kinds of poor eating as there are people. Insofar as investigating all eaters is obviously impossible, we must be satisfied here with a survey of some of the more common poor eating patterns and assumptions. To simplify matters, I call these poor consumptive patterns "maladaptive eating." They cluster around two extremes. At one extreme are deprivation practices, in which eaters deprive themselves (or are deprived by others or extenuating circumstances beyond their control) of adequate nutrition or certain foodstuffs. At the other extreme are gluttonous practices, by which eaters overeat for conscious or subconscious purposes. Simplifying maladaptive eating into these two broad categories of course suppresses the complexity such eating habits entail. Still, appreciating such extremes is heuristically valuable as it will enable us to better situate adaptive eating practices and assumptions.

The terms *maladaptive eating* and *adaptive eating* deserve some attention. While they are frequently used in medical and scientific arenas, they also have deep and old connotations. As I will show throughout this book, civilizations throughout history have worried about healthy eating. Those that have grown and prospered have done so in part because they identified healthy consumptive patterns; others shrank or disappeared altogether when their eating behavior no longer was sustainable. This holds true as well for individuals. When persistent, maladaptive eating patterns often compromise a person's ability to mature, thrive, and even procreate. Additionally, each person's dietary pattern adjusts throughout life. What was once food, like breast milk, may no longer suffice or entice. Bodily needs also change, from, say, pregnancy or exertion or age. Eating to meet those ever-shifting needs is thus part and parcel of adaptive eating. Adaptive eating is as evolutionarily advantageous for individuals as for a species. A central goal of this book is to discern, from ancient times to now, what constitutes adaptive eating.

Part II, "I Eat Therefore I Am," disaggregates the various components of eating. First: the eaters. Chapter 3 wonders about the noun, the subject who eats. Oddly, few scholars focus on the fact that we humans are just like every other living creature: we are eaters of the world. Next is the eaten, the object consumed. Much has been written about food, and in chapter 4 I organize this growing conversation into a few broad genres. This better situates my own project as an example of eating ethics. In chapter 5, I turn to eating itself, the verb that eaters do with and to the eaten. Here the physiology and philosophy of metabolism come to the fore.

Part III, "Eating Well," examines the centrality of eating to human existence. From the very moment we emerge from the womb, all humans clamor for sustenance, and this biological fact is reflected in religious stories about the primordial beginnings of humankind. Yet the eating these religious resources promote is not unbounded; it is circumscribed. They teach that eating should be moderated. Chapter 6 explores moderation through ancient philosophical ideas of temperance and contemporary scientific studies of satisfaction. Indeed, the very notion of being sated is core to this book's project. Eating to be sated is not a new idea, however. Ancient religious traditions insist that eating well means eating less than what one can hold physically, as well as eating more than nothing and not too little to sustain us. I explore these ideas and what they might mean in a modern context in chapters 7 and 8.

Part IV, "I Eat Therefore I Am Tasteful," homes in on three features of eating well. Certain tastes, such as sweets, salts, and fats, have come into disrepute in the contemporary food environment primarily for their deleterious impact upon human health when consumed without constraint. Savoring (chapter 9) these critical components for human nutrition requires appreciating their potential for health and for harm. Sacrificing (chapter 10) unbounded consumption of these and other tastes is both biologically and religiously called for. Such restraint, chapter 11 argues, contributes to personal as well as communal well-being, for it enables sharing and commensality: restraint cultivates eating together.

Part V concludes the book by stepping back from these arguments from religion, philosophy, and physiology to wonder about broader implications and applications of the call to eat until one is satisfied. Some may contend that this suggestion to eat less than what our contemporary food environment encourages is impolitic, too onerous for a few, dismissive of eating's complexities, or the like. Others may worry it will encourage those who already eat too little to continue to do so. Some may hold that this proposal glosses over the many injustices built into the fabric of the modern food industry, from farms to abattoirs to food deserts to school lunches.

Others may deride this project because it does not directly address the elephant in the modern public health room: obesity. Anti-obesity literature is what is needed, they may say, not yet another book about eating. Yet one might wonder about the efficacy of that genre and its tact. It construes obesity as the culprit needing capture, a problem that requires solving. Although probably unintentionally, such conversations about obesity depict the obese themselves as culprits and problems, as troublemakers wreaking havoc on economies, homes, even the environment. Anti-obesity approaches also misplace cause and effect insofar as they construe obesity as the cause of so many ailments, personal and social alike.

A different approach would understand obesity as a symptom of deeper, more complex conditions and decisions. So often obesity is a consequence of circumstances rather than the cause of them. Speaking in negative terms about the consequences does little to nothing to change the conditions giving rise to them in the first place.

Instead of being anti-obesity, or only about that, this book's tack is pro-health. A pro-health approach labors to identify ways of thinking and behaving that promote health and prevent obesity—not ways to react to obesity and mitigate its serious and complex problems. In brief, this book proposes an integrated, proactive—or adaptive—strategy toward eating well.

Eating well can hardly be prescribed at a general level with much accuracy. This is because each eater is unique, with idiosyncratic bodily needs and palate preferences. What I can and should eat will be peculiar to me; what you can and should eat will be different. Eating well must be individualized; a prescribed eating regimen may endanger me—or you—if it is maladaptive to our unique bodies. What satisfies me will probably be different from what satisfies you. So instead of putting obesity and its related maladies at the fore, this book concerns you—the eater—no matter your size or situation. This is a book about you who eat.

# 2

# DEPRIVATION AND GLUTTONY

*More people have succumbed because of the pot than [because] of famine.*

—Babylonian Talmud, *Shabbat* 33a

When the Apostle Paul thanked the citizens of Philippi in Macedonia for sending gifts while he was ill, he reiterated the importance of being vigilant even when doing good. Regarding those people who mistake earthly things for ultimate goods, Paul said, "Their end is destruction, their god is the belly."[1] These belly worshippers do wrong in two ways. On one level, presuming stomachs are gods is nothing short of idolatry. On another level, belly fixation can lead to deadly outcomes. Theological and physiological dangers accompany belly worship. In more modern terms, being so consumed *with* one's belly is to be consumed *by* it.

Let us orient ourselves to healthier—and holier—guides.

Before I explore what those healthier ways of consuming might be, we need to appreciate the ways in which we so frequently become consumed by our own bellies; how our assumptions and behaviors about ourselves and specifically about ourselves as consumers are often deleterious, if not dangerous; and how our eating practices damn and damage. That is, we need to identify problematic eating so as to understand why better eating is needed in the first place.

Let me reiterate that my concern here is not morphology, is not about body shape and size. Some might wonder, "How does the fat [or the ultrathin] body come to signify immoral behavior?"[2] This is a provocative question. It is also potentially dangerous. It can lead one to conclude that those whose bodies are unreasonably beyond the range of normal are not just guilty of immoral behavior but are immoral in their very being. It also reinforces popular notions that those whose bodies are abnormally fat or thin deserve the maladies that accompany those conditions. They get their just desserts, so this line of thinking goes.[3]

In my view, such inquiries and thinking are misguided. Though body shape, size, and weight may be influenced—and influenced a great deal—by personal choices, especially habitual ones, they are also impacted by forces beyond personal control. Geography and climate, zoning laws, socioeconomic situation, war and other exogenous stressors, available foodstuffs, hormones and metabolic flora, and more influence body size and health.[4] This is not to absolve everyone of any and all responsibility for their body's shape, size, and well-being. Nor does it assume in a crass manner that the obese "are guilty [of gluttony] and thus owe the rest of us an apology or an explanation for having offended."[5] Same for the ultralean. Size is neither crime nor offense.

Rather, we recognize that morphology is often already late, indicative as it is of perhaps poor choices but also of disadvantageous circumstances well beyond personal control. To put it succinctly, neither excessive fatness nor excessive thinness is simple; their causes are complex, and placing blame solely on the persons whose bodies are excessive ignores or belittles those complexities (and probably both).

Consider children, for example. For the most part, children eat what they are given; they do not choose or control much of what they consume, when, how, where, with whom, or why. Moreover, according to a commentary in the *Journal of the American Medical Association*, especially in the United States, children eat in a highly pressurized environment in which "ubiquitous junk food marketing, lack of opportunities for physically active recreation, and other aspects of modern society promote unhealthful lifestyles in children."[6] Children are vulnerable to these larger socioeconomic environments as well as the smaller ones constructed by their parents and families. All these factors can be obesigenic, that is, contributors to excessive weight gain in children.[7] Should overweight and obese children be held morally accountable for these larger and complex influences well beyond their control? I would hope not.

Consider other harms caused to children who are exposed to such obesigenic influences. In addition to gaining more weight than would be normal for growing and maturing bodies, overweight and obese children can suffer "immediate and potentially irreversible consequences, most notably type 2 diabetes," and these almost inevitably lead to macrovascular and microvascular diseases, permanent pancreatic ß-cell malfunction, or death—all of which dramatically reduce life expectancy.[8] Reactive and invasive procedures like bariatric surgery could be used for short-term impact on body weight and size. This approach, however, addresses primarily the symptoms of larger and earlier maladaptive patterns, especially of consumption. They do not solve the underlying problem but merely "kick the can down the road."

A different solution put forward in that *JAMA* commentary is to acknowledge that overweight and obese children, vulnerable populations that they are, need state protection. The state can override parental rights so as to protect the interests of the child. We already do this in regard to other forms of abuse and neglect: children are removed from those dangerous environs to avoid immediate and cumulative harms. An argument could be made, then, that children suffering life-threatening obesity are similarly subject to abuse and/or neglect and their immediate and chronic harms rise above a threshold that mandates state intervention: they should be removed from such environs for their own protection. Undoubtedly this proposal is controversial, impractical, and perhaps illegal in many situations. Yet it raises a critical question: If childhood obesity is so dangerous, why is more not being done to prevent it rather than react, post facto, to its myriad maladies and costly, lifelong consequences?

This brief discussion of childhood obesity is meant to demonstrate that body weight and size is often beyond personal control. Similar observations could be made about the extraordinarily thin. Often those who are waif-thin have underlying health problems that include and stem from dietary patterns. Body size and weight are thus more often *symptoms* of earlier conditions and patterns of consumption. They are the *results* of many actions, circumstances, and, yes, choices.

Unfettered logic would perhaps lead us to address the many prior or earlier causes of extreme weight. Yet strong arguments that appeal to economic and political motivations undermine such reasoning. For example, there is much money to be made from the obese, as evidenced by the repeated failures of fad diets (they will try another), bariatric surgery (we can cut again), and medicines for chronic life-threatening conditions (caring for but not curing a condition guarantees a lifetime purchaser).

Similarly, it can be argued that the extremely thin can serve as enduring sources of profit for plastic surgeons, dieticians, and pharmaceutical companies. Political arguments often disfavor proactive initiatives toward extreme weight. Given the American commitment to individualism and autonomy, it is far easier to say in public that people should be free to eat whatever they want (or not) and whenever they want than it is to advocate constraining consumptive choices or proactively instituting healthier conditions. According to such logic, it is better to fix a problem once it arises than to prevent it in the first place.

This book takes a different and perhaps less popular tack. Instead of obsessing about the very bodies that frequently indicate long-standing maladaptive eating practices and thus offer late "solutions" that are in fact not solutions at all, I focus on that earlier central contributing factor to problematic weight: eating itself. Paying more attention to inputs than outputs will shift the conversation away from reactive stances to ones that are more proactive. It acknowledges that no two bodies are alike: each requires unique nourishment, and because of this, no singular prescriptive diet could ever be appropriate for all bodies. Some bodies require more of this or that, others less. Eating well is an individualized enterprise that takes the peculiarities of each body into account. The actual or perceived weight or shape of our bodies matters less than what we put into our bodies, how, and why. While in fat studies this idea is often conveyed as "health at any size,"[9] I will speak more about "eating well at any size." In so many ways, size is all but irrelevant: I will speak about eating well.

## MALADAPTIVE EATING

As extremely overweight and underweight bodies are often (though admittedly not always) evidence of not eating well, I should clarify what is meant by maladaptive eating. Physiologically speaking, orderly or adaptive eating for the most part accords with metabolic needs, that is, with the needs of the body. In contrast, maladaptive eating is "eating . . . no longer confined by metabolic needs."[10]

Whether ordered or disordered, there are three interacting systems that influence a body's eating, and all have a brain component. *Homeostatic*

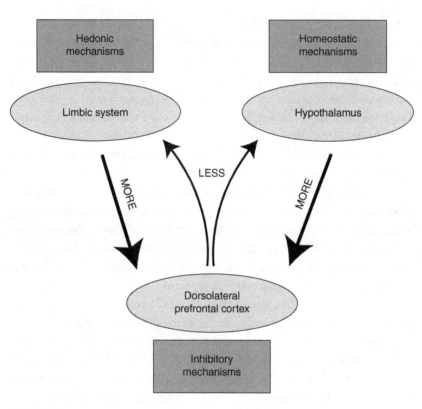

**FIGURE 2.1**

Adaptive or ordered eating includes three interacting mechanisms, each with its own brain component.

*mechanisms,* guided in large part by the hypothalamus, encourage eating to replenish depleted energy. We eat after rigorous activity to replenish the energy our body exerted and to once again achieve internal equilibrium, or homeostasis. *Hedonic mechanisms,* by contrast, angle for food rewards, which are signaled through the limbic system. Sweet foods are particularly powerful dopamine-generating sources; because they are intensely pleasurable we are all but driven to consume them. *Inhibitory mechanisms* constrain eating; they operate through the dorsolateral prefrontal cortex. As will be discussed in greater detail in chapter 5, when a person eats adaptively or in an orderly manner, these three systems interact in such a way that the body's energy needs are met (homeostatic), enjoyment is experienced (hedonic), and the meal is stopped when the body and brain are satisfied that enough of the right stuff has been consumed (inhibitory).

These interactions are troubled in maladaptive eating. Chronic overeating, or hyperphagia, for example, may override inhibition. Hyperpalatable foods—those that are high-sweet and/or high-fat—often trick the homeostatic system into thinking that more should be consumed to meet energy needs. Much research has been and continues to be done on how and why maladaptive eating occurs at all and recurs in certain individuals and populations. Though that ample and rich literature need not be rehearsed here, a few general points do merit highlighting.

## SO SAD

Maladaptive eating certainly includes issues of quantity. In today's food environment, the Standard American Diet (SAD) encourages eating too much as well as too little. As I will discuss in subsequent chapters, in recent decades meal sizes have ballooned. Serving sizes, too, have grown: candy bars and drinks are some of the most obvious indicators of this trend. Mindlessly we purchase and consume quantities of food that far exceed our bodily needs because in large part such sizes are what is available in stores, restaurants, delis, ballparks, and the ubiquitous drive-thru. Recent studies have shown that what contributes most to overweight and obese conditions is not meal frequency but meal or portion size.[11]

Conversely, SAD's message to consume too little comes predominantly yet not exclusively from the diet industry. Strategies to pursue weight loss (again, a reactive goal) invariably include limiting the consumption of fats, calories, carbohydrates, salty foods, snacks, desserts, or whatever the author of a diet construes as the culprit for causing excessive weight gain. Eliminate these evil items from your fare, and ideal body weight and shape will be yours, or so these diets promise. However, study upon study show that these sorts of diets fail more than 80 percent of the time.[12]

Another maladaptive feature of SAD regards quality. The kinds of food SAD promotes are highly processed, which invariably decreases or eliminates altogether nutritive elements of ingredients. While processing certainly enhances shelf life, improves packaging possibilities, and obviates transportation concerns, it also makes these foodstuffs convenient and cheap. But their relative pervasiveness and cheapness do not make them good to eat.

The contemporary food environment also encourages homogeneity, even monotony. Processed food in one corner of the country will probably be exactly the same in another corner. Regional variation is rare. This geographic or spatial homogeneity is also true in time. So-called seasonal processed foods are seasonal not because their component ingredients are seasonally limited but predominantly for marketing reasons. (Think of gingerbread mix so abundant near Christmas time and all but absent in other seasons.) On the whole, SAD encourages us to eat the same foods all the time with very little seasonal variability, reinforced by restaurants and stores that offer the same fare all the time in every location. (Think of franchises.) Such constancy of supply across time and space necessarily curtails the food quality available for us to consume.

A third way SAD troubles our eating regards frequency. We eat maladaptively when we eat too frequently or infrequently. After decades of pressure, the modern food industry has successfully created a new American pastime: snacking. Food and beverage companies ingeniously developed, marketed, and sold stuff to consume at all times of the day and night, regardless of what one is doing otherwise. Portable containers continue to proliferate to enable us to eat and drink most anywhere anytime. Architecture, too, facilitates purchasing yet another thing to consume. Consider how drive-in and drive-thru restaurants pockmark the landscape and, inside buildings, how take-out counters and cue-control mechanisms quickly shuffle customers to order, pay, and retrieve mass-produced foodstuffs. The ease with which we can access consumables does not mean, of course, that what we consume nourishes. On the contrary, even in this food culture of apparent bounty, increasing evidence demonstrates that malnutrition abounds.

The quantity, quality, and frequency of our eating practices could instead be adaptive; that is, they could promote our personal and collective health. Unfortunately, SAD demonstrates that we have manipulated each of these facets of our food environment to such an extent that our eating has become risky, if not dangerous. In so many ways, SAD makes maladaptive eating the norm.

SAD's unwitting promotion of maladaptive eating is not a unique phenomenon. Many civilizations around the world and throughout history have promoted consumptive patterns that were maladaptive, undermining personal and population-wide health. On the other hand, as far as I know, all civilizations have also urged good eating by warning against eating that transgressed certain norms, especially religious norms. As I will discuss shortly, harmful eating has long been identified as a problem and strongly discouraged.

## DEPRIVATION

To be sure, restrictive diets vary. Some restrict when one eats, while others restrict what one eats. Some, for example, fixate on certain ingredients or foods and mandate avoiding them. This is perhaps most famous in the general Islamic and Jewish prohibitions against eating pig. The vegan diet of Jains includes the avoidance not just of all animal products but also of plant foods that require the destruction of the plant itself (e.g., carrots, ginger, onions, and other tubal vegetables). This is to dietarily reinforce the Jain commitment to *ahimsa*, or nonviolence. Modern, secular diets similarly identify culprit foods or ingredients and prohibit or severely limit their consumption.

Some diets do both: they restrict what one eats for a certain time period. Take Lent as an example. During this forty-day period leading up to Easter that includes self-denial, prayer, penance, and charity, Christian believers are to refrain from consuming certain foods to mimic Jesus's fasting in the desert, especially on Ash Wednesday and Good Friday. Another is Ramadan, a month-long observance by Muslims during which they consume neither food nor drink during daylight hours. Like Lent, Ramadan is a lengthy period for spiritual reflection and self-control. During Yom Kippur, Jews are to refrain from eating and drinking for twenty-five hours, from just before sundown until just after sundown the next day. This solemn holiday spurs critical self-analysis and repentance.

Hindus observe numerous fasts that are typically a day long to honor specific deities. These frequently entail severely restricted food consumption and sometimes complete abstinence from all food and drink.

Though these religious holidays restrict consumption temporally, it would be inaccurate to describe them as diets per se. They are fasts; diets, by contrast, are consumptive regimens meant for longer durations. Fasts, physiologically speaking, last eight to twelve hours, long enough for food and drink to be fully digested. Observing such religiously sanctioned lengthy breaks between meals requires not putting food and drink into one's mouth. This is one reason the meal concluding, say, Yom Kippur, is called "breakfast": it breaks the fast one held. The morning meal in many cultures is called breakfast, for as one sleeps one also fasts. At least this is so in theory; many people snack long into the evening, and some wake in the middle of the night for a repast. Such practices put into question whether their "breakfast" is a misnomer.

Still, insofar as fasting figures significantly in religious calendars, we can conclude that these traditions celebrate the rigors of fasting. It stands to reason religions would not commend fasts as much as they do were fasting something easily done; simple tasks hardly prove or stimulate conviction and commitment. One illustration of this logic is the exemption Judaism provides to those who are pregnant or sick: they are explicitly *not* enjoined to fast because doing so can be risky.[13] In fact, because religions frequently describe fasting as something difficult, it is viewed as a powerful expression of faith. Pope Leo the Great said as much in a sermon in the fifth century: "We order to you this fast of December . . . because it conforms to piety and to justice to render thanks to God after having received the fruits of the earth and to offer him the sacrifice of mercy with the immolation of fast."[14] On this account, inducing one's hunger expresses gratitude for the divinely provided bounty one typically consumes.

Yet not all fasts are the same. The prophet Isaiah worries about fasting that is done for the wrong reasons:

[The Judeans cried:] "Why, when we fasted, did You not see? When we starved our bodies, did You pay no heed?" [Isaiah answered:] Because on your fast day you see to your business and oppress all your laborers!

Because you fast in strife and contention, and you strike with a wicked fist! Your fasting today is not such as to make your voice heard on high. Is such the fast I desire, a day for men to starve their bodies? Is it bowing the head like a bulrush and lying in sackcloth and ashes? Do you call that a fast, a day when God is favorable?[15]

In his view fasting is not just meaningless but mean when done for improper reasons and with misdirected antics. Such a fast would be empty socially and theologically; it would be a profoundly hungry hunger. The rabbis later debated what to call someone who fasts just for the sake of fasting. Some thought this individual was a sinner, while others held that this person was holy or pious. One rabbi concluded that a dog should devour this person's meal because he or she did not deserve a meal to break an ill-conceived and poorly performed fast.[16] The absence of consensus about fasting for fasting's sake suggests it enjoys no blanket religious imprimatur.

Regardless of how fasts are perceived and evaluated, perhaps their most significant feature is that they are highly regulated.[17] From time immemorial, religions have gone to great lengths to stipulate when fasts should be done, by whom, where, how, for how long, and for which purposes. Take the Qur'an's instructions as an illustration:

O you who have believed, decreed upon you is fasting [just] as it was decreed upon those before you [so] that you may become righteous. [That is, fasting for] a limited number of days. So whoever among you is ill or on a journey [during those fast days]—then an equal number of days [are to be made up]. And upon those who are able [to fast, but with hardship]—a ransom [shall be paid by you as a substitute:] of feeding a poor person [each day]. And whoever volunteers excess—it is better for him. But to fast is best for you, if you only knew.[18]

Fasting is serious business and needs to be controlled in shape, size, and duration; exceptions are identified and preferences proclaimed. Regular, pro-adaptive eating is—must—bookend religiously sanctioned fasts. Fasts are not meant to be interminable.

Haphazard fasting would not only go against religious authority and doctrine; it would endanger fasters themselves. Fasting done well need not be maladaptive. Indeed, it can enhance one's well-being in addition to one's spiritual health; according to the Qur'an, fasting correctly improves one's righteousness, for example. We therefore distinguish fasting from other forms of consumptive deprivation that typically are known today as eating disorders.

Eating disorders take different forms. Restricting consumption on a wholesale basis is often called anorexia. The Greek roots of this term are *an*, meaning "without," and *orexis*, meaning "appetite" or "desire": the anorexic is—or tries to be—without appetite. Identifying the origins or causes of anorexia is now a robust enterprise, involving behaviorist, biochemical, sociocultural, psychodynamic, and other schools of thought. Regardless of the approach taken to explain anorexia, all perspectives agree that it is a maladaptive eating strategy.

Bulimia is another maladaptive eating strategy. Whereas anorexics refrain from or severely limit putting foodstuffs into their mouths at all, bulimics induce vomiting after they consume. In so doing they prevent their bodies from digesting and extracting nourishment from what has been ingested. Their hunger (*limos*, in Greek) becomes ravenous, like an ox's (*bous*, in Greek). When done chronically, bulimia wreaks havoc on a body by depriving it of essential nutrition as well as causing it to endure the violence of regurgitation time and again.

A related maladaptive restrictive practice is binge eating, when more is eaten in a discrete period of time than would otherwise be eaten. That binge eating is a restrictive eating disorder might seem odd, but binge eaters for the most part drastically control and limit their consumption and only in certain instances let themselves eat to nausea. This kind of sporadic consumption is disinhibited, compulsive, and impulsive. Binge eaters report such feelings as panic, depression, and loss of control. Stress and severe dietary restrictions often trigger binge eating.[19]

Not all binge eating evidences a disorder, however. Some binge eating occurs in culturally fabricated situations, such as eating competitions. Such events—a modern invention if there ever was one—include assessing how much a person consumes in a particular time frame and involve audiences that enthusiastically watch competitors grab and gulp as much as possible as quickly as possible. Whether it be a spaghetti-eating

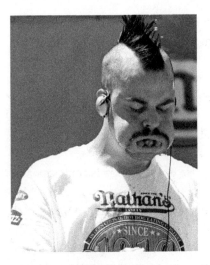

FIGURE 2.2

A competitor at a recent Nathan's Hotdog Eating Contest.

event at a picnic, a county fair pie-eating contest, or beer guzzling in a pub, such competitions thrill audiences near and far.

The most famous binge-eating competition today is probably Nathan's annual Hotdog Eating Contest, held on the Fourth of July.[20] Ever since 1916 the company has hosted an eating contest of its highly processed product. In recent decades the increasing popularity of this event has necessitated a feeder system, literally: competitors must qualify at regional events around the country before convening for the finals in Coney Island, New York. The race is on to see who can eat the most hotdogs and buns in ten minutes. In addition to ESPN televising the event live to a national if not international audience, the winner receives trophies and other paraphernalia as well as digital immortalization on the company's website. Such eating competitions have spawned Major League Eating, "the world body that oversees all professional eating contests."[21] While it would be tempting to say that since eighty or so competitive eating events in a given year occur in the United States, sponsored binge eating is peculiar to the U.S. eating landscape, but this would be inaccurate. Eating competitions and competitors are increasingly popular in Canada, Japan, Australia, and the United Kingdom.

In recent years in the United States, another deprivation diet has emerged that severely restricts consumption. While not intended to be maladaptive or contrary to bodily thriving, in its severest forms it is. Called orthorexia (*orthos*, Greek for "straight," "proper," "correct," + *orexis*, "desire" or "appetite"), it is the unhealthy obsession with healthy eating. Orthorexics become consumed about their consumption. They worry about the quality and quantity of their foods to such an extent that their idiosyncratic eating concerns override many other aspects of their lives, which not infrequently leads to social isolation and, ironically, nutritive deficits.

A major contributing factor to the rise of orthorexia is contemporary culture's fascination with thinness and health. When studies emerging nearly weekly about the benefits of this food or the dangers of that nutrient and the outcomes of certain kinds of exercises are coupled with the overall marketing ethos in which thinness is portrayed as valuable, it is no wonder many feel pressure to eat a certain way to look a certain way. This is precisely one of the problems of orthorexia and many other kinds of maladaptive deprivational eating practices: they predominantly respond to external cues.

## GLUTTONY

A whole other class of maladaptive eating strategies is associated with excessive consumption. These excessive ways of eating are more pervasive in the contemporary food environment than restrictive ones. Here, surfeit consumption by quantity, quality, and frequency is the norm. Gluttonous eating is nothing new, obviously. That people ate until they had glutted their guts was a phenomenon famous enough for Aristotle, all those thousands of years ago in the fourth century BCE, to describe them thus: "To eat or drink whatever offers itself till one is surfeited is to exceed the natural amount, since natural appetite is the replenishment of one's deficiency. Hence these people are called belly-gods, this implying that they fill their belly beyond what is right. It is people of entirely slavish character that become like this."[22] Remember that the Apostle Paul said those who mistake earthly things as ultimate goods, like worshipping their own bellies, pursue their own destruction. Aristotle here seems to worry that belly worshippers become enslaved; they lose their freedom even as they freely stuff themselves. In his view, the civilized person does not indulge to such an extent.

Indeed, Aristotle distinguishes between the self-indulgent and those who are merely fond of something, like certain foods. Those who are fond of this or that food take delight "either in the wrong things, or more than most people do, or in the wrong way." One can be fond of unhealthy food, for example, or fond of consuming too much of something, or fond of consuming something in a way that compromises one's flourishing.

Self-indulgent persons, by contrast, exceed in all three ways. They delight in the wrong things, in consuming more than most people do, and consuming them in the wrong ways. The indulgent also "craves for all things or those that are most pleasant, and is led by his appetite to choose these at the cost of everything else." When they fail to get what they so desire, such individuals feel extraordinary pain, more pain than most people do when their desires for this or that food are frustrated. The self-indulgent thus pursue the pleasurable at all costs: they eat too much of the wrong food and in the wrong ways precisely because the very act of consumption is so enjoyable to them.

Insofar as the indulgent person seeks pleasure for its own sake, this person's eating would be unregulated and uncontrolled. In Aristotle's view, the indulgent person's pleasure is, by definition, unreasonable, and given his preference for reason, such eating is eschewed. Reasonable eating, by contrast, is not devoid of pleasure but is reasonably pleasurable.

Interestingly, Aristotle does not specify precisely what the wrong food is. Rather, he wants to identify the category of the self-indulgent as those who delight in pleasures more than those pleasures are worth.[23] In this way he provides philosophical acknowledgment of both orthorexia (the unhealthy indulgence in healthy foods) and gluttony (the unhealthy indulgence in unhealthy foods). He believes both kinds of excessive consumption are unreasonable, and because of this they are undesirable. Humans ought not eat unreasonably; they should eat according to the dictates of reason, that is, with some semblance of control, and derive reasonable pleasure from such controlled consumption.

Like Aristotle, St. Benedict of Nursia (c. 480–550 CE) had a similar concern about self-indulgence. Benedict was so worried about it that he instituted a rule for Christian brethren that continues to be followed by many monastic communities to this day. Regarding the measure of food to be eaten in a given day, dinner, he says, should consist of two cooked dishes, with seasonally available fresh fruit and vegetables, and some bread. "Above all things, however, over-indulgence must be avoided and a monk must never be overtaken by indigestion; for there is nothing so opposed to the Christian character as over-indulgence, according to Our Lord's words, 'See to it that your hearts be not burdened with over-indulgence.'"[24] Benedict invokes Jesus's teaching that indulgence entraps, distracts, and undermines readiness for the moment when believers will stand "before the Son of Man."[25] On Benedict's account, surfeit consumption is more than contrary to idealized Christian character; it compromises a central goal of Christianity itself, which is to be ever-ready for Jesus's second coming and one's own redemption. Indulgent eating is thus simultaneously maladaptive (it can cause indigestion not just after one meal but chronically, not to mention all the other related maladies) and theologically dangerous.

For St. Thomas Aquinas in thirteenth-century Italy, gluttony is most definitely theologically dangerous. Using Pope Gregory I's teachings on gluttony as background, Aquinas identifies five types:

- *Praepropere* (Hastily)—eating too soon or at an inappropriate time
- *Laute* (Sumptuously)—eating extraordinarily costly foods
- *Nimis* (Too much)—eating an excessive quantity
- *Ardenter* (Greedily)—eating too eagerly or ardently
- *Studios* (Daintily)—eating foods too elaborately prepared

On Aquinas's account, the glutton who spurns God so as to enjoy the pleasures of gluttony has committed a mortal sin, whereas the glutton who enjoys the pleasures of gluttony but does not spurn God has committed only a venial sin. Either way, gluttony is a capital vice, which leads to other vices; for all these reasons, such extreme eating should be eschewed.[26]

The early modern German philosopher Immanuel Kant (1724–1804) also weighs in on excessive eating. When stuffed with food, he says, an individual "is in a condition in which he is incapacitated, for a time, for actions that would require him to use his powers with skill and deliberation."[27] Consuming to the point of stupor obviously "violates a duty to oneself," he contends. Worse, it renders one inhuman: "Gluttony is even lower than that animal enjoyment of the senses, since it only lulls the senses into a passive condition and, unlike drunkenness, does not even arouse imagination to an active play of presentations; so it approaches even more closely the enjoyment of cattle."[28] Gluttonous consumption is bovine, not human.

What Kant emphasizes in "On Stupefying Oneself by the Excessive Use of Food or Drink" is not that excessive consumption brings about bodily harm, because this is obvious and can be easily counteracted with arguments in favor of well-being and comfort, which would "establish only a rule of prudence, never a duty." Rather, Kant wants to make a stronger argument against gluttonous consumption. Insofar as excessive eating stupefies, it "depriv[es] oneself (permanently or temporarily) of one's capacity for the natural (and so indirectly for the moral) use of one's powers."[29] It is a moral duty *not* to eat indiscriminately—not because it would lead to bodily harm but because such bodily harm compromises one's moral capacities. Bovines cannot be moral in the ways humans are or should be moral.

We should note that neither Aristotle nor Benedict nor Kant mentions anything about body size. The shape of a human body is of less concern than a person's eating. For all three, excessive eating is worrisome because it compromises or obviates one's reason, one's theological readiness, and one's ability to be moral—not to mention one's bodily integrity.

Since eating excessively as an eating strategy harbors a full range of dangers, stuffing oneself silly is an activity one should not do on a regular basis. Yet feasting is not to be disparaged and discouraged wholesale so that one would never eat excessively. For millennia, proto-humans and early humans ate what they could scrounge and gather. If by luck they came across a dead animal that had not yet rotted, they would consume it and take advantage of its dense proteins and fats. Our bodies thus evolved to survive and thrive on calorically restricted eating strategies that were only occasionally interrupted with intense feasts.

In time, cultures and religions around the world came to regulate abundant consumption just as they do fasts. Such feasts populate calendars, but only periodically. Consider, for example, Passover, a springtime

banquet during which Jews eat foods symbolic of slavery, retell their liberation from servitude, and consume great amounts of food during the
evening's celebrations. The feast of Easter, around the same time as Passover, looms large in the Christian calendar, as does the feast on December 25 celebrating the birth of Jesus (as well as of Mithra and the Roman
holy day of Saturnalia), which traditionally has been the most extravagant
meal in the Christian calendar, against which all others are measured.[30]
Eid-al-Fitr concludes the month-long fasting period of Ramadan for Muslims. Though traditions vary around the Muslim world, Eid is typically an
all-day consumptive affair with countless dishes and courses. Nonreligious feasts also regularly occur in cultures. In America, at least, Superbowl Sunday, the Fourth of July, and Thanksgiving are prominent in the
secular calendar. Such overly large meals are designed to be special. They
are meant to be unusual consumptive experiences overladen with religious and secular dimensions. Their significance—in size if not in spiritual impact—would diminish were all others meals similarly large.

Though this concern is perhaps not what animates him, Kant nonetheless articulates a worry about frequent banqueting. In his view, banquets tempt intemperance. Conversations at them are limited to one's
immediate neighbors, so they cannot be as morally stimulating as
smaller dinners with fewer people in which conversation could last a
long time. He therefore wonders "how far moral authorization to accept
these invitations to intemperance extend."[31] Insofar as feasting promotes
recklessness and irrationality, Kant recommends feasting only occasionally. Were Kant alive today, he would probably find repulsive the modern
food culture in which nearly every meal is treated like a banquet, with
copious food and drink, eaten with distracted and distracting companions, if any at all.

Kant's issue—as it is for many—is not feasting per se but feasting continuously, which is gluttony. The viciousness with which ancient traditions and early moderns like Kant attacked gluttony—declaring it not
just a vice but a sin—is understandable given their socioeconomic circumstances. They lived in times when scarcity was prevalent and superabundance nonexistent. In the words of William Miller, a professor of
law, gluttonous consumption in that kind of economic order was a kind
of "murder or a kind of criminal negligence, like drunk driving is for

us. . . . Eating was a zero-sum game. The more you ate the less someone else did. And any ingestion beyond what was necessary for the maintenance of life was an act of injustice."[32] In Miller's account, gluttony in times of scarcity was a heinous crime worse than stealing; at base, it was murder. Though Miller's may be a hyperbolic interpretation, the point remains true today: gluttony in a superabundant context is a damaging, maladaptive eating strategy for individuals and communities.

## SEEING MALADAPTIVE EATING

The complexities of eating at the extremes are perhaps better expressed in images than words. Consider, for example, two engravings composed in 1563 by the Flemish engraver Pieter van der Heyden (c. 1530–c. 1575). He worked in the booming port of Antwerp, which in the first half of the sixteenth century was the second largest and most economically vibrant city in northern Europe. It was a time of great religious upheaval: Luther's 1517 protests in Germany produced waves of reforming movements throughout Europe, Antwerp included. Political upheaval was the norm, culminating with the Eighty Years' War (1568–1648) for Dutch independence from Spanish rule. Relative abundance, instability, and insecurity thus characterized van der Heyden's context.

His *La Cuisine Grasse* (The Fat Kitchen) is the more famous of the two engravings. It shows a table piled high with haphazardly stacked dishes of hardly eaten foods, most of which are made of fresh animals. Two children cram scraps from the floor into their mouths. Three pots sputter on the fire; a spit with a pig and fowl drips sauce and fat into a puddle, itself lapped up by a rotund cat. The dog chomping on a sausage at the bottom and the puppy biting the starving vagabond with the bagpipe at the door who is being pushed and kicked out demonstrate that living animals are as obese as the people. A robust baby can hardly suckle for lack of space on the indifferent woman's lap. A necklace of sausages enwraps a man, cross-eyed from surfeit consumption, stuffing yet another bite into his engorged face. Another obese man with a sausage in his bulging belt and his face bloating from gas or indigestion—or perhaps indifference— gesticulates rudely toward the vagabond, as if to push him farther away

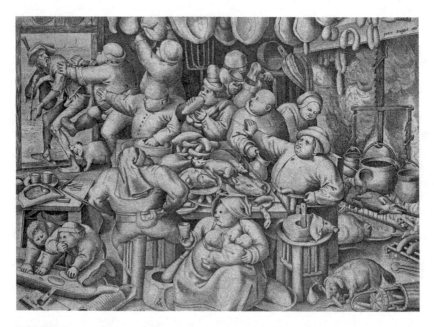

**FIGURE 2.3**

Pieter van der Heyden, *La Cuisine Grasse*, 1563. http://images.metmuseum.org
/CRDImages/dp/original/DP825757.jpg.

from the as yet uneaten bounty. To add insult to injury to the vagabond,
even as food literally drops from the table, more is being cut from a hanging cheese just near the door. No one looks at anyone else except those
who look with disdain and disgust at that poor vagabond. Civility in such
an eating environment has been obliterated. Without saying a word, this
image powerfully contends that habitual excessive consumption contorts
persons and even society itself.

The other picture, *La Cuisine Maigre* (The Lean Kitchen), depicts in
somewhat gruesome detail what happens when deprivation becomes the
norm. Here five people apparently share from a single dish, and none appears hearty or hale. This may be because their food is just a mess of mus-
sels served with bread and hardly anything else. The paucity of the table
reflects the fact that their larder is all but empty, a sign indicative of ongoing food insecurity. The impoverishment is total: a bald and muscle-
wasted child buries its head in a pot to lick its sides; an emaciated baby is

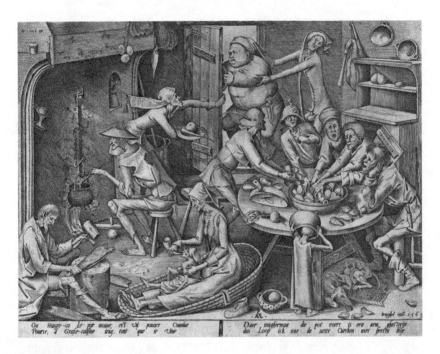

**FIGURE 2.4**

Pieter van der Heyden, *La Cuisine Maigre*, 1563. http://www.metmuseum.org/art
/collection/search/392426.

tenderly fed some liquid concoction through a funnel held by a malnourished woman with shriveled breasts; a single pot steams on the fire tended
by a bone-thin cook. Even the dog hiding under the table hungrily licks
empty shells so to somehow nourish her whimpering whelps. A man sits
by the fire beating slabs of probably salted meat to tenderize them for
whatever meager nutrition they may hold. Though the overweight man
at the door desperately tries to leave, the same vagabond who had been
kicked out of the other house (note the bagpipe hanging on the wall) here
squeezes the man's arm as if to bring him in. Another slender figure vig-
orously holds the door open and offers the large man an apple and a carrot. Does the large man flee because he fears the vegetable and fruit, or
might he be uncomfortable that such poor folk are so keen to share
their meager fare while his own obese folk shared only cruel indifference, or might he wonder whether cannibalism is their intent?

Sharing is one thing; taking one's fair share is another. A man at the table apparently begrudges his neighbor's two-handed grab into the common pot.

At one level, van der Heyden portrays the dangers of chronic eating strategies at the extremes. Both deprivation and excess undermine personal health, just as they compromise civility. Beware, he seems to say: extreme eating is maladaptive for one and all. Because they are dangerous they should be avoided. Do these pictures provide a historical lineage to the *JAMA* proposal to extract children from homes in which extreme dietary practices are the norm?

Not all is black and white, however. Van der Heyden's pictures suggest ambivalence about extreme eating. In a gluttonous context, the vulnerable of society—children and breastfeeding women, for example—could have access to the excess of the excessive. The dregs, waste, and crumbs produced by surfeit eating practices can become potential fare for those who do not have access to the table, literally or figuratively. Of course, not all who are hungry have access to such unwanted bounty: the vagabond is forcibly being removed from the scene. Still, as Miller observes, something in gluttony permits "some redistributions from rich to poor—paltry, but redistributions nonetheless."[33]

In a similar vein, restrictive dietary regimes are not merely exercises of deprivation, of cutting off and out. Consider the eagerness with which the thin men try to include and entice the large person to join them. They exhibit a rare kind of hospitality. They acknowledge that even the overly large can be hungry; all deserve a place at the table, even if the offered fare is meager. At least at this table a person may encounter an interlocutor, someone who acknowledges one's very existence.

Little romanticism emerges from van der Heyden's depictions of eating at extremes. He embraces neither gluttony nor deprivation; he holds them at a distance to observe their many demerits and few benefits. When viewed together, his pictures promote avoiding both kinds of maladaptive eating strategies since they are disadvantageous—to oneself, one's family and friends, and even one's society. Other eating strategies surely exist that are in and of themselves advantageous and pro-adaptive, that are as nourishing for one as they are conducive to human flourishing for many. Clarifying at least one of these strategies is at the heart of this book.

## SHALL WE EAT?

If belly worship is dangerous, if being so consumed by one's food is disadvantageous, would being the opposite be any better? Jesus taught his disciples that anxiety about such earthly matters is unnecessary: "I tell you, do not worry about your life, what you will eat, or about your body, [or] what you will wear. For life is more than food, and the body more than clothing."[34] Some might interpret Jesus to mean that one should not care *at all* about one's eating. If it is theologically fine to consume anything in any quantity at any time, then it stands to reason that it should be physiologically fine. However, such reasoning backfires.

Others might think that Jesus is suggesting that one should care not to eat *at all*. This would be folly, too. Eating is a human necessity. (More about this in subsequent chapters.) Without any nourishment humans would die; we would be unable to manifest God's will—or anyone else's will—in the world. Such would be a self-defeating eating strategy.

Instead, as Jesus says, strive for the kingdom of God and God's righteousness—and food, drink, and clothing will be provided.[35] In this way Jesus says it would go against Christian teachings to be either overly anxious about one's eating or overly lax: both extremes would be maladaptive and transgressive in equal measure. Holy and hearty eating exists between such extremes.

# I EAT THEREFORE I AM

*An organism becomes a food only when created as such.*

—David Goldstein, *Eating and Ethics in Shakespeare's England* (2013)

# 3

# THE EATER

*The universe is nothing without the things that live in it,
and everything that lives, eats.*

—Jean Anthelme Brillat-Savarin, *The Physiology of Taste* (1999)

veryone eats. This much is obvious. Less clear is what it means to be an eater. What does it mean to consume our world, literally? Why do we incorporate into ourselves that which is not us? What does it mean to devour and drink and stuff ourselves? Why is it that we so often forget the fact that we are eaters?

This last question should perhaps come first. Even as we stuff ourselves, we so rarely recognize ourselves as eaters, as consumers of the world. Why? Why do we consistently skip over this regular feature of our existence?

One reason we so frequently dismiss the reality that we are eaters is morphological: physically we cannot see ourselves eat. We are blind to our own eating because our mouths are beyond the horizon of our eyesight. As our eyes are situated above our cheeks and nose and lips, we cannot gaze upon that orifice into which we shovel our food and drink. Our own mouths exist and operate beyond our eyesight; what happens therein is a mystery to us.

Because we cannot directly see our own mouths, we easily forget that we ourselves are eaters. When we think of eaters as such, we typically think of other people; we can at least observe them putting morsels into their mouths. Many of us who are parents or care providers actively put food in the mouths of others, mouths that are right there before our very eyes. With their mouths so available for us to observe and stuff, no wonder we think that they—and not we personally—are eaters.

So when conversation turns to eating and eaters, we tend to think about others more than ourselves. They are eaters, not I. Whatever problems or imbalances or issues there might be in regard to eating, other people should be the ones who need to pay attention, not I. This approach displaces concern by ignoring the fundamental fact that each of us is an eater. By diminishing the importance eating has for each of us, this perspective compromises our personal and collective flourishing. Lest we continue eating blindly, and harmfully, we need to reflect on the fact that we each are eaters, consumers of our world.

## DEAD EATERS

We should not be surprised that we do not usually think of ourselves as eaters. Thinking about ourselves has an ancient lineage. Western society has thought long and hard about what it means to be human. A curious feature of this heritage is that for the most part, it is devoid of the human body and perforce of the eating body itself.

The fifth-century BCE Greek philosopher Socrates famously argues in Plato's *Phaedo* that philosophers should not deign to dabble with "the so-called pleasures connected with food and drink."[1] The human body only distracts the truth-seeking mind with its fickle appetites and needs. Philosophers, Socrates seems to say, would do well to abandon their bodies; indeed, they should even be hostile toward them. Such aversion to the material body, to that which decays and passes, will only help philosophers attain greater clarity of forms and eternals. Escape from fleshy existence should be sought, not feared. At its extreme, thinking is best done when dead.

Socrates's student Plato says as much: "True philosophers practice dying."[2] Just over a century later, Epicurus, the philosopher whose name is now associated with pleasure, and pleasure of the palate in particular, also endorsed the idea that death ought not be shunned but embraced. On his view, one should derive pleasure from *ataraxia*, equanimity or tranquility, and this is best done by living quietly and modestly (*lathe biōsas*) and not by pursuing extraordinary pleasures of the palate.[3]

That philosophers should be indifferent or have antipathy toward their bodies was amplified by perhaps the most influential philosopher on Western thinking in the modern era: the French intellectual René

Descartes (1596–1650). A committed rationalist, Descartes derided empiricism's view that truth can be derived from physical evidence. For him, thinking is the source of what matters; truth emerges from within the mind, not outside it. *Cogito ergo sum*—I think, therefore I am— became his watchword.[4] To think is to exist.

For Descartes, the perceived and experienced world is just that. The world is mediated by the senses, and what is sensed is ultimately mediated by the mind. The body merely relays to the mind what it can, and the mind is the final grasper of reality. The Cartesian body is essentially an organic machine composed of strings and levers, joints and beams, conveying information from exogenous stimuli to the mind. Once given the body's data, the mind is free to range as far as it can deduce and imagine. Whereas the mind is a powerful, willful unity, the body is a passive concoction of this and that.

This dualist or mechanistic perspective understands the human body as hardly more than a piecemeal collection of interchangeable parts. Just as with today's complex machines, if something in the body no longer functions as it should, the solution is simple: go in there, take out the malfunctioning piece, insert a new one, put it back together, and press restart . . . ad infinitum. If the body is truly and only a machine, what makes it work can rightfully be likened to fuel. Eating, in the Cartesian view of things, funnels fuel into the belly, where it undergoes biological combustion, if you will, which itself produces actionable energy and waste byproducts. The body both transmits this energy wherever the biological machinery needs it and excretes whatever the machine cannot use. Like fueling a vehicle, eating is purely utilitarian, a necessary activity to get from A to B, from now to then. Ideally, of course, eating fuels the highest and purest of all human endeavors: thinking.

In this worldview, the thinker is not an eater as such but a kind of biological tank. Tanks have caps, though, a limit beyond which fuel will spill out and be wasted. One thus does not eat the world as much as opens one's belly for the mind's fuel. This formulation construes the person as a passive receptacle, all but indifferent to the very act of being filled. Indeed, filling this tank to capacity seems logical insofar as that inserted fuel would inevitably be transformed into useful energy, especially for thinking. In other words, fill the belly to the brim to empower the brow.

For a variety of reasons such views of the body and fueling it have come to dominate Western thought and practice. We invariably speak of ourselves as composites of bodies *and* minds or souls.[5] Material and ethereal, we operate with dualist assumptions about the nature of human existence. A clear indication of this assumption is the definition of death. Life, we so frequently say, ends when the soul departs the cooling body. Of course medical professionals use a more technical and biological definition that revolves around irreversible brainstem and/or cardiovascular death. But the point remains: the mind's functioning is one thing, and the body is another.

Dualism presumes our bodies are in part, if not wholly, ultimately disposable. Even though our beloved minds need working bodies to think, dualism views bodies as machines. Since their pieces are replaceable, bodies are, at base, fungible. Like a lawnmower, a body can be turned off, manipulated, partially replaced, and switched back on at will—as long as the singular mind remains unaffected. Our bodies can be left in sheds to rest until we need them next. Hence the rise of cryopreservation, of deep-freezing bodies and/or heads for some hoped-for future in which bodies can be thawed, rejuvenated, and cared for, if not cured outright. Though some transhumanists are working hard to make possible the separation of mind and body and their ultimate reconnection, the reality remains that our minds cannot operate or survive without being attached to vibrant bodies.

Herein lies the rub with dualism. While most machines could wait indefinitely in the proverbial shed until being restarted, organic bodies cannot. All biology decays, especially when it is not laboring for its own preservation. If our bodies were truly machines, as Descartes imagines, they would stop working the moment food leaves the belly, just as a car sputters to a stop when its tank empties. But as we all know, our bodies do not immediately cease functioning when our stomachs become empty. The body begins to extract energy from itself by drawing on its stores of fat; when the stomach is empty, the body cannibalizes itself, if you will. Some might argue that this is still a machine-like function as those fat cells are the body's batteries. There is a key difference, however. A machine's battery may house energy additional to what is extracted from fuel in its tank. When the machine consumes the battery's energy, the battery remains just as bulky and heavy as it ever was. Fat in an organic body, by contrast, shrinks and ultimately can disappear as it deploys energy back to the larger organism. These fat "batteries" self-eliminate.

This points to an even larger problem with the dualist conceptualization of humankind. Just as the body is not a machine, food is not only fuel. A machine is a passive recipient of the fuel poured into it. The machine burns the fuel or otherwise transforms it into energy and waste, and then transfers the energy as needed. The organic body similarly brings food into itself, "burns" it, produces waste and energy, transforms energy for physical and psychical purposes (or stores it as fat), and excretes waste. So far it seems bodies and machines are the same and that food is fuel and fuel is food.

But there is a critical difference: fuel never interacts with the machine itself. It never becomes part and parcel of the machine, in contrast with food and the human body. Whereas fuel passes through the machine, food becomes the body. Its energy and nutrients are absorbed by the body itself. The body incorporates food. Food literally becomes the body that consumes and metabolizes it. Through metabolism, bits and pieces of the body retire and are escorted out along with unabsorbed eaten things. Food becomes body and body becomes waste. Fuel never becomes the machine itself.

Were we truly Cartesian machines, what we put into our mouths would not, for all intents and purposes, impact our bodies as such; it would only pass through us. We could then easily consider ourselves not as eaters but as users who put the world's energy into use for our peculiar psychical endeavors, much as machines use energy for their mechanical activities. Like machines, we would be essentially detached from the world, as indifferent to it as it would be indifferent to us except in regard to energy (and waste) transfer. Our relation to the world would be in terms of equations: so much in means so much out.

Since concerns about input and output dominate this kind of worldview, what matters most for existence (I am reluctant to say *flourishing*) is quantity of energy flow. Thinking of ourselves as bodily machines may seem odd, but this image is alive and well in today's weight-obsessed culture. Those diets and exercise regimes that fixate on "calories in and calories out" operate with a Cartesian notion of the body and its relation to the world. They construe the body as a machine requiring so much caloric fuel that is then transformed into action by the body's burning it. If one were to desire losing weight, one would need to ensure that one's caloric output surpassed one's caloric intake; conversely, if one wanted to gain weight, one would need merely to consume more calories than one expends. Boiling it down, we would be biological machines, simultaneously passive and vulnerable to simplistic equations of fuel in and energy out. Our health, indeed our very vitality would ride upon the calculations, permutations, and ratios others tout as holistic, as the next sure thing for peak bodily and—more important—mental performance.

If we are honest with ourselves and consider the ample and growing evidence around us, we have to admit that thinking about ourselves this way has failed us.

## LIVING EATERS

Socrates ironically drank himself to death, albeit with hemlock, and Descartes was just wrong. Thinking is done only while alive. Our bodies are not machines, and we are not impervious to the world. We do not just use energy, nor are our body parts infinitely replaceable. Our minds are not separable from our bodies, nor can our bodies exist apart from our minds. We are not all but dead, dualist entities; we are living, singular eaters.

The Dutch philosopher and theologian Baruch Spinoza (1632–1677) took Descartes to task for favoring the mind and belittling the body. However powerful the human mind may be, Spinoza insisted, its omniscience pales in comparison with God's. The relatively puny human mind cannot know the human body in its totality as it might know a machine whose pieces it made and can distinguish with absolute certainty and ease. The human body is much messier and murkier than Descartes describes. In Spinoza's view, the body comprises many "individual [parts] of different natures, each of which is highly composite," such as fluid, soft, and hard materials, and these materials are continuously affected by external bodies in various ways. "The human body, to be preserved, requires a great many other bodies, by which it is, as it were, continually regenerated."[6] Full comprehension of this ongoing interaction between self and world requires perfect knowledge, and only God can know that much. Thus, Spinoza says, whatever we can know about this complex relationship between external materials and the elements of our bodies will necessarily and at best be inadequate and imperfect.

While Spinoza dislikes Descartes's hubris, his critique centers on the Cartesian notion that our bodies are mechanical puppets beholden to the mind. On Spinoza's account, there cannot be a radical separation between mind and body, nor can human existence be apart from the world. Rather, mind and body are united and should be understood as such. Nourishment is meant to ensure that this complex unity can thrive, enjoy, and contemplate:

> To use things, therefore, and take pleasure in them as far as possible—not, of course, to the point where we are disgusted with them, for there is no pleasure in that—this is the part of a wise man. It is the part of a wise man, I say, to refresh and restore himself in moderation with pleasant food and drink, with scents, with the beauty of green plants, with decoration, music, sports, the theater, and other things of this kind, which anyone can use without injury to another. For the human body is composed of a great many parts of different natures, which constantly require new and varied nourishment, so that the whole body may be equally capable of all the things which can follow from its nature, and hence, so that the mind also may be equally capable of understanding many things at once.[7]

Eating, for Spinoza, is no purely utilitarian enterprise; it involves aesthetics as well as ethics.[8] It is an intricate, all-encompassing activity, unlike a machine's merely burning fuel. We live in a complex dependency—an interdependency, really—with our environment, with "new and varied" pieces of it passing into us and of us into it.

Even though Spinoza makes no bones that understanding this intricate relationship exceeds his gambit, he challenges us to understand it better, for our very vitality and flourishing depends upon it. To begin with, it would be best for us to acknowledge ourselves as eaters insofar as we are biologically bidden to bite the world around us. Because we frequently snatch a piece of it for our personal consumption, we would do well to appreciate—by which I mean think deeply about—this fact of our own, individual existence as consumers of our world. I am just like every other self out there: I too am an eater.

Of course, this is not news. Even as the ancient biblical teacher Kohelet bemoaned that all appears vain, he also observed that each person's existence requires being an eater: "Who will eat and who will enjoy, except for me?"[9] Outsourcing this vital requirement for life is impossible. Insofar as each person lives, each must be an eater.

Eaters eat in different ways, to be sure. What bothered Kohelet was that many people lived and ate according to the mistaken notions that the stuff of this world has ultimate meaning, that the accrual of stuff is life's purpose, and that enjoyment now can endure beyond death. Such material hedonism and the eating it engenders lead only to vexation, sickness, and wrath.[10] Mindless, selfish consumerism is as physically damaging as it is theologically degenerate. It is venal and vain.

Kohelet instead promoted a different way of understanding oneself as a consumer in and of the world. Insofar as each person is an eater, it would be best to understand oneself as an eater alongside others, not against others, as do material hedonists. Meaningful human existence means to be eaters who enable others to eat as well or, as I will discuss further, eaters who enable others to eat well as well. This is achieved not by eating at the extremes. On the contrary, eating for meaningful human existence is done by consuming only what is in one's God-given portion.[11]

## EATERS OF THE WORLD

Brillat-Savarin famously quipped, "Dis-moi ce que tu manges, je te dirai ce que tu es"—Tell me what you eat, I will tell you what you are.[12] Just as one cannot be unless one eats, so too one's eating conveys one's identity. Your eating communicates your values, commitments, convictions, and circumstances. How you attend to your own bodily needs and appetites says a great deal about how you think about yourself, the world, and others.

As noted, eaters of the world exist alongside other eaters of the world. The pithy maxim "Eat or be eaten" highlights that there are multiple, coexisting consumers in the world. Acknowledging that we are not the only eaters *of* the world *in* the world may seem so rudimentary as not to merit mention, yet it is a fact that has inspired profound philosophical reflection.

Levinas, for instance, meditated a great deal on eating and what it means to be an eater. He argues that to be an eater requires attending both to one's own hunger as well as the other's hunger. He makes this claim in part by meditating on the terms *gero, gerere, gessi, gestus*, Latin for "carrying" and "bearing." From that root come such terms as *exaggerate* (to pile up), *belligerent* (one who wages war), *register* (to list or record), even *suggestion* itself (to bring up). It also links to eating: *ingest* (to bring within), *digest* (to break apart what is held), *egest* (to defecate). More, it connects to fecundity and specifically to maternity in the word *gestation*.

What does it mean to gestate, to carry another within oneself? How does gestation connect with being an eater? Levinas wrote that "gestation of the other in the same" is the primal—indeed, the exemplary—*gesture* (how the body is carried) of hospitality.[13] This is because to gestate another in oneself is to feed the other within. Even more profound, one feeds the other within despite oneself. Gestation and hospitality obviate voluntarism: the will is immaterial and irrelevant. In gestation, the idea of willfully giving nourishment to another is unintelligible because it cannot be otherwise. The hosting body feeds the guest, and the guest consumes the host—and this is the essence of life. Christianity encapsulates this interrelationship in the sacrament of the host or Eucharist, which I will discuss in a later chapter.

To gestate—to host or to be hospitable—is as much about feeding as it is about eating. As Levinas says elsewhere, this kind of being for another despite oneself is "to take the bread out of one's own mouth, to nourish the hunger of another with one's own fasting."[14] Eating and feeding are inextricably linked, just as sustaining the self and nourishing the other go hand in hand. Maternity and hospitality, Levinas seems to say, are indistinguishable gestures.

To be hospitable is to give nourishment to another, to enable another to enjoy filling a basic need: hunger.

Let's pause for a moment on hunger. All eaters get hungry. This is as true for microscopic bacteria as for humans. Hunger signifies a creature's very creatureliness. Ethereal entities like angels and deities never hunger because they are, by definition, immaterial. As hunger is an exclusively biological phenomenon, Levinas argues that it is "constitutive . . . of the materiality and the great frankness of matter."[15] Hunger constitutes life.

Hunger, for Levinas, has two facets. The romantic side of hunger laments that magical stories, smells of food, or sounds of clinking money do not mollify hunger's unremitting pangs. The unreal is impotent, and realizing this makes hunger worse. The other side of hunger despairs of its own incessant, material existence. This biological reality of hunger paradoxically inspires one to be interested in both one's own hunger as well as others' hunger. Because my hunger wants and needs to consume what is beyond me, my hunger is a kind of transcendent experience. This is no generic ethereal transcendence, however. I know that nothing magical can mollify my hunger, and because I know this about myself it must also be true about your hunger. I can be certain that you, like me, need something real to eat. "The new transcendence," Levinas concludes, "is the certainty that nothing can deceive the hunger of the other man."[16]

Even though I know for certain that only real food will attend to your and my own hunger, who should have first dibs? Enabling another to enjoy eating is curious because the other's enjoyment means nothing if one has not also and already enjoyed the nourishment one now provides. Levinas says, "One has to first enjoy one's bread, not in order to have the merit of giving it, but in order to give it with one's heart, to give oneself in giving it."[17] Most anyone or anything can provide food, as the natural world does all the time to those who reach out and grasp what's around them. Such offering or giving of food acquires meaning only if that food has already been partially consumed and enjoyed.

This gesture of offering food not wholly consumed yet fully enjoyed is the marker, par excellence, of the moral subject.[18] Again Levinas: "But giving has meaning only as a tearing from oneself despite oneself. . . . And to be torn from oneself despite oneself has meaning only as a being torn from the complacency in oneself characteristic of enjoyment, snatching the bread from one's mouth. *Only a subject that eats can be for-the-*

other."[19] Only the one who eats can be a moral subject, can be oriented toward another and labor for another's well-being. Only eaters can simultaneously nourish another, and in this way eaters can be for-the-other. Eaters nourish others with real, not magical food.

This is not to say that eating is the sole mechanism by which moral subjecthood is constituted. On the contrary, eating is merely the first hoop through which all must jump en route to becoming a moral mortal: "The morality of 'earthly nourishments' is the first morality, the first abnegation. It is not the last, but one must pass through it."[20] David Goldstein, a contemporary scholar of Renaissance literature and consumption, explains the significance of Levinas's argument this way: it is eating that "teaches us about our complex relationship to objects, in preparation for an acknowledgment of other beings."[21] Eating is not merely a hedonistic, solipsistic endeavor done in isolation. It is not an act whose exclusive goal is homeostasis. To be an eater is to be in a reflexive, iterative, and instructive relationship constantly renegotiated and complicated by others whom we may, or perhaps may not, eat yet whose own hunger we must confront even if only unconsciously. We may say that how we attend to our relationship with our own eating, as well as with the fact that we are inescapably eaters alongside myriad other hungry eaters, necessarily embodies and conveys our very ethicality.

To be a living eater *of* the world means to be an eater *in* the world. It is to coexist with other eaters who are similarly radically dependent upon the world for nourishment. We see their hunger even as we experience our own; we see them eating, though we cannot observe our own masticating mouths. We eat the world just as they eat the world. Being an eater is inherently an ethical feature of biological existence. We can ill afford to ignore, belittle, or be blind to this fact.

# 4

# THE EATEN

*Eat food. Mostly plants. Not too much.*

—Michael Pollan, *In Defense of Food* (2008)

Before we can talk about eating food we would do well to appreciate how we have come to talk about food.

Eaters eat something. This something cannot be just anything, however. It has to be something eaters can take into themselves and, via the powers of digestion, transform its elements into usable energy. The eaten must be a certain kind of thing that revitalizes biological organisms. It must simultaneously be

- not the organism itself;
- in the world around the organism yet not so far away that it cannot be grasped and eaten;
- ideally not poisonous;
- composed of components beneficial to the consuming organism.

The eaten defies simplification. Calling all things eaten *food* disguises the fact that all things eaten are not food.[1] The contemporary food writer Michael Pollan makes this point in his *In Defense of Food*. He finds that much of what we humans eat today is not food per se but foodstuffs, concoctions of chemicals manipulated to trick and tease our senses and digestive tracts. Though we may enjoy these foodstuffs, and though many have fats and carbohydrates that have some nutritional value, on the whole they are not necessarily things that nourish and revitalize our organisms. Rather, increasing evidence demonstrates that what passes as foodstuff has deleterious effects on us, individually and collectively. Some foodstuffs outright poison us.

Not only do many foodstuffs endanger those who eat them, but how they are produced, packaged, and sold is no less damaging. According to the contemporary American writer and environmentalist Wendell Berry:

> The passive American consumer, sitting down to a meal of pre-prepared or fast food, confronts a platter covered with inert, anonymous substances that have been processed, dyed, breaded, sauced, gravied, ground, pulped, strained, blended, prettified, and sanitized beyond resemblance to any part of any creature that ever lived. The products of nature and agriculture have been made, to all appearances, the products of industry. Both eater and eaten are thus in exile from biological reality. And the result is a kind of solitude, unprecedented in human experience, in which the eater may think of eating as, first, a purely commercial transaction between him and a supplier and then as a purely appetitive transaction between him and his food.[2]

We eaters eat in exile, displaced many degrees from our "food." The theologian and ecologist Norman Wirzba echoes this point: "When food is reduced to a commodity and we to consumers, it is inevitable that our primary concern will be that food be inexpensive, convenient, and in plentiful supply. The ease of exilic eating and the facility with which the unjust and destructive dimensions of our food economies can be hidden and ignored make it likely that we will learn to prefer the state of exile, forgetting, perhaps even forsaking, our food-providing home."[3]

Berry, Wirzba, and others make clear that we can ill afford to ignore the fact that how we develop and package food distances us from what we eat—literally in our markets and literarily in our words. Thankfully, the complexity of our current food system and its many problems are increasingly coming under scrutiny by journalists, academics, activists, politicians—and even consumers themselves.

## TALKING OF FOOD

What do we talk about when we talk about food? In recent decades, various conversations have emerged on food and food's impact on us as individuals, collectives, civilizations, and even the world writ large. These conversations fall into three major camps or genres, each with its strengths and limitations: food ethics, dietetics, and eating ethics.

*Food ethics* is concerned predominantly with how food moves from farm to fork. It investigates such issues as farming practices like irrigation and pesticides that impact the environment, migrant labor and unions, transportation and logistics, manufacturing of foodstuffs, additives and preservatives, marketing, distribution and retailing, farm subsidies and food stamps, urban food deserts and restaurant placement, not to mention all the issues surrounding animals, including husbandry and genes, vaccination, housing, feeding, culling, transporting, slaughtering, packaging, and animal waste—and there's *a lot* of waste.[4] Attention is given to such themes as social justice, sustainability, and food safety. Many alternatives have been suggested to improve the development and movement of food from its genesis to its ultimate location, which is the plate in front of me. I call this genre food ethics insofar as one of its central goals is to inform, if not alarm, so as to influence how we think, make policy, and ultimately exercise our wallets.

Consider as a gripping illustration Michael Moss's 2013 Pulitzer Prize–winning book, *Salt, Sugar, Fat.* Through his investigative journalism, he exposed the ways some industries generally and certain companies specifically scheme and manipulate ingredients to make their products ever more attractive, if not addictive. His study garnered a lot of attention in part because it was written as though it were a witch hunt, uncovering how these villainous corporations eagerly take advantage of gullible consumers through devious production and marketing strategies. Though Moss stopped short of calling American eaters innocent, he nonetheless suggested they were participating in an insidious industry that makes certain shareholders and corporate leaders wealthier and the population at large unhealthier.

The second kind of conversation is focused on *dietetics.* This genre subdivides into the *descriptive* and the *prescriptive.* Regarding the latter, chefs, nutritionists, celebrities, hunters, gardeners, and many others prescribe diets they tout as the best way to, say, manage or lose weight, prepare and consume particular ingredients or nutrients, fast or feast, take advantage of seasonal local produce, practice a particular cuisine, promote libido, manage and even reverse health problems, and more generally ensure healthy longevity. Sometimes based on scientific evidence but oftentimes not, many of these programs combine self-help advice, motivational psychology, structured regimens, surveillance mechanisms to watch and measure consumptive patterns, and, of course, recipes. These idealized diets are promoted on food channels, documentaries, and talk shows, inspiring practitioners and converts. They flare up in popular culture, driving demand for certain ingredients and instruments, classes and memberships. Eventually they fizzle and fade as the next fad diet rages onto the scene, promising just like the old ones to fix America's everexpanding waists, haywire hormones, and faulty veins.

One encouraging example in this genre is Rip Esselstyn's Engine 2 diet. A former world-class triathlete and firefighter, Rip promotes a plantstrong diet that promises to reduce weight, improve bloodwork numbers, and offer tasty meals. Drawing on cutting-edge scientific evidence of the disaster that is the Standard American Diet and of the benefits a wholeplant diet provides, Esselstyn aims to convince and inspire people to transform their otherwise destructive consumptive habits to this particular wholesome one. His is a multipronged approach, including books (with recipes, of course), blogs, documentaries, immersive "seven-day rescue challenges," weekend retreats at a family farm, and more.[5]

The more descriptive side of dietetics identifies cultural patterns of producing, cooking, and consuming foodstuffs. This is what many call foodways, a rich and long-standing field of scholarship that investigates how people create cuisines, develop and inculcate certain culinary attitudes, and practice commensality of eating at the same table. Unlike prescriptive dietetics, these descriptive projects are predominantly written by scholars using anthropological, historical, social, religious, and economic tools, usually studying a particular community's, region's, or historical period's relation to food. Often they reflect upon food's complex roles in shaping social relations and the symbolic dimensions of certain ingredients, foods, cooking, and consumptive practices.

Clifford Wright's *A Mediterranean Feast* is an impressive history of culinary cultures surrounding the Mediterranean basin and illustrates well the scholarly approach to foodways. He describes his project as "a book of food, and a book about food, informed by a history of the environment, an ecology of the Mediterranean, the lives of ordinary people, the importance of trade and transit, the development of town and capitalism, the beginnings of the nation-state, and the familiar story of great men and wars. But it is also a book about food in history, and about history. It attempts to challenge some notions we have about the food we eat, where it comes from, and how it developed."[6] Wright traces how culinary patterns and specific dishes emerged and evolved. The book is more than a traipse through food history, though; it includes over five hundred recipes adapted for the modern kitchen to "show the full range of culinary ingenuity and indulgence, from the peasant kitchen to the merchant pantry."[7]

Though both kinds of dietetic literature focus on food, their purposes are not the same. The study of foodways labors to identify the features and boundaries of particular populations' ways of considering, using, and consuming food. Central to these kinds of projects is the question of authenticity, for instance, What is authentic Corsican cuisine? How did Elizabethan England eat, in contradistinction to eras before and after or in other lands at that time? Diets, by contrast, seek compliance and allegiance. Whereas the study of foodways explores authenticity and identity, diets desire obedience.

Missing in all these discussions, however, is me: the individual person who eats. Though diets prescribe idealized regimens, they do so with limited sensitivity to my particularity, my idiosyncratic bodily needs and preferences. For the most part, diet advocates work hard so I know the ins and outs of the proposed diet, where to purchase key ingredients, how to cook in particular ways, when and what to eat and how much. Such programs direct my attention outward, toward their plan for the food that I am to eat. Or, sometimes, these programs instruct me about human metabolism, physiology, health, illness, and aging. But they teach me all this biology by speaking of generic humankind, as if I am no different than everyone else. By making me look away from myself, these diets orient me to know their diet more than my unique body. I can lose sight of myself because of the diet.

Examining foodways, by contrast, quietly puts me into question by juxtaposing me, rhetorically, against some other group that I may or may not be a member of; it does not study me and my eating as such. These projects look at a given community, analyzing its rules and practices, such as kashrut or hallal, and often situates it within larger socioeconomic, geographic, and philosophical contexts. Though some foodways scholarship in religious studies explores theological treatments of eating bodies, rarely do they integrate discussions of the physiology of eating.[8] For the most part, I—this living, eating body now—am absent in foodways studies.

The first genre, food ethics, by contrast, urges me care to about how food gets to my kitchen, to wonder generally about the nature of what I eat, whether and in which ways it is natural at all. Yet food ethics rarely meditates on me as an eater or on what eating itself might mean. Its central concerns are the effects of food and eating in the aggregate, not my personal experience of them as such or what they mean to me. Food ethics is less concerned about how and why you and I use our mouths when eating than about how and why we open our wallets. This genre on the whole eclipses the fact that we are biological eaters in favor of seeing us as socioeconomic political actors.

To be sure, discussions in food ethics and dietetics are enlightening and constructive. Yet in them the eater as such has frequently been misplaced, aggregated, or ignored altogether. Food also is variously treated by these genres. For some, the eaten is supposed to be this, not that, taken in this way and not that way. For others, the eaten bespeaks boundaries, identities, commitments. And for still others, the eaten is a symptom or evidence of larger civilizational issues like hubris, greed, and scientism— the belief that science, and chemistry in particular, is food's foundation and controlling its chemicals is of paramount concern.

All genres agree, however, that food is where personal, social, scientific, political, economic, religious, environmental, and historical issues are at play. What food means, how it is conceived and manipulated, how it is served and consumed are questions fraught and complicated and continuously renegotiated, consciously or not. For these reasons and more, such genres contribute a great deal to contemporary thinking about food and eating.

For the most part, however, these approaches speak of food and eating from the outside. Their contributors tell us what is and is not food, what are appropriate amounts to prepare and how. They dictate to us what to eat, when, and why. Often they tell us the impact our food has on others (humans, animals, the environment, the economy, etc.) as well as on our own (generic) bodies. They inform us about what food does *to* us, but only on occasion what food does and is *for* us.

I propose a third genre to complement these discourses that homes in on the eater. This genre takes seriously the one who actually masticates, metabolizes, and meditates on eating. This genre focuses not on the movement of food from farm to fork but on the movement of food from plate to palate to physique. Specifically, it explores how the very fact and act of eating constitutes the eater. Instead of paying attention to what someone else says I should or could eat, or what a potential food or food-stuff does to others, or what some food or regimen might do to a generic body, this approach takes the eaten—what I actually eat—seriously. It considers what food and eating do *for* me, not just what they do *to* me. It speaks of food and eating from within the perspective and experience of the eater, which is every one of us. By encouraging us to understand food and eating from the inside by learning how to appreciate our internal cues—by teaching us to learn and shape our unique relationships with food and eating—this genre augments the more external perspectives championed by the other literatures.

I call this kind of discussion *eating ethics*. Its ethics are not confined to philosophical schools of consequentialism (where the ends justify the means) or deontology (where an act is moral to the degree it complies with a preconceived duty or principle). Rather, its ethics lie in the truth that eating is in and of itself an ethical enterprise, no matter how one thinks about it. Just as eating is an inherently ethical enterprise, food itself is similarly an ethical construct: it is socially defined and defining, as demonstrated by conversation in dietetics. Food is also an ethical construct because it directly impacts me the eater and the eaten, not to mention the contexts in which this eating occurs, inclusive of humans, other sentient creatures, the environment, and more, as food ethics readily explains.

In brief, unlike the other genres, eating ethics considers simultaneously the eater, the eaten, and the very relation between them: eating itself. Eating ethics is not a more perfect conversation than the other ways of talking about food and eating. It is a way of talking about food and eating that situates each eater at its core—a core so central to food that to dismiss it is to miss the point of the whole conversation. Eating ethics thus complements food ethics and both kinds of dietetics.

## TAKING OF FOOD

One might think that food is only a thing that is taken into the mouth. Food is this, to be sure, but it is so much more. It also includes that which the body takes into itself. Nearly two hundred years ago Brillat-Savarin made this point: "What is meant by food? *Popular reply*: Food is everything that nourishes. *Scientific reply*: Food is all those substances which, submitted to the action of the stomach, can be assimilated or changed into life by digestion, and can thus repair the losses which the human body suffers through the act of living. Thus, the distinctive quality of food consists in its ability to submit to animal assimilation."[9] What we take from the external world and blindly shovel into our mouths—whether solid or liquid or some non-Newtonian gooey substance like ketchup or whipped cream—does not stop at our tongues. The mouth is only the beginning of food's journey through our internal worlds: food passes beyond the tongue into the esophagus that automatically transports it down to our stomach, where it is churned in an acidic soup to expose its elemental nutrients for easy absorption into the body as it moves along the small and large intestines and is ultimately expunged from the body through the colon, liquids being evacuated via the kidneys and bladder. I will discuss the physiological processes of eating and metabolism in greater detail in chapter 5.

To be blunt, food at the mouth is not food for long. What goes in our bodies undergoes radical changes before it exits our bodies. Compare this to the mechanical view of the body as championed by Descartes. Fuel, as in a car, endures but one significant change: combustion transforms the liquid into gases, and the necessary expansion required for those gases is converted into mechanical energy, as well as heat and exhaust. Fuel thus becomes usable energy, dissipated energy transferring heat away from the engine block lest the machine's integrity be compromised, and waste. As noted earlier, energy captured by an engine makes the machine run, but it never becomes the machine itself. It is never incorporated; fuel does not inform the machine's body. Through metabolic processes, however, food becomes heat and waste, as well as the body itself. This waste, which I will discuss in the next chapter, is not only residue of what was recently eaten; it includes pieces of the consuming body that now need to be escorted out. The stuff that exits the body is simultaneously both less than and more than the food taken in. Exhaust, by contrast, hardly ever includes bits of the machine that are no longer needed.

Food is rarely static either as a thing out there in the world or as a thing consumed. Minerals aside, before it reaches any mouth, food is organic and thus subject to decay. Although we consider ourselves omnivores, all-competent consumers of the organic world, we do not eat just anything or everything.

This holds true for all creatures. All living things must eat, yet not all living things in the world are food for all. The physician and philosopher Leon Kass observes that food simultaneously relates and differentiates living things: "Something is *as* food only to another being—one that almost universally belongs to a different species."[10] This is a difference of kind, not degree. Rare is the creature that eats conspecifics, members of its own species. We eat what is not us.

The very category "not us" is admittedly vast and vague. No creature—not even humans—eats all things existing in that "other" category. Some entities are outright poisonous: they would be an eater's last meal. Other things are just not available, living in climes the eater does not. Some entities may be edible but are not preferred; an eater has tried them before and would rather not eat them again. A few items are unappetizing from the get-go because an eater has been trained to dismiss them. Some things disgust eaters for reasons that transcend culture. And some foods were once readily consumed with gusto but are no longer because tastes change.

Breast milk is but a quick illustration. Mammals, humans included, suckle for a while and eventually outgrow the habit or are weaned. On the whole, human babies self-regulate. Because they detach when sated, overfeeding a breast-fed baby is all but impossible. Underfeeding and even hyperregulating breast-fed babies is easy. This fact about neonates' capacity to self-regulate their consumption of what is "not them" must mean that self-regulation is evolutionarily adaptive. It would be a leap in logic to argue that since people become maladaptive eaters later in life their dysregulated eating is learned behavior. It could be that people naturally outgrow the self-regulation inherent in us as infants, or that such self-regulation is linked specifically to eating at a nursing breast. On the other hand, an argument could be made that contemporary food cultures and pressures disabuse people of their innate self-regulatory consumptive practices and replace them with other kinds of consumptive directives and models. Put differently, the naturally occurring internal cues for eating that even babies live by can be and often are displaced for manufactured external cues. I will talk about this more in chapters to come.

If mother's milk transitions from being food to nonfood for an individual human, other foods may similarly shift between the eaten and the not, and vice versa. This shifting is idiosyncratic, unique to each individual. Take mushrooms, for example. When younger I found the smell of cooking mushrooms to be nauseating, and were I to eat them I often vomited. Today I can tolerate mushrooms, raw and cooked, though I do not voluntarily order, say, *tagliatelli e funghi*. The primary reasons for my initial aversion was sensorial: mushrooms smelled and looked ugly to me; I found their slippery texture repulsive, and their taste made me gag. In time such reactions faded, and though my preference is for other kinds of foods, I will now eat mushrooms.

This is not true, however, of other foods. A younger me used to eat all sorts of land animals. I thought it was normal to buy, prepare, cook, serve, and consume chicken, duck, cow, lamb, and all sorts of sea creatures. But experience and education changed my attitude toward consuming animal flesh. I came to find such foods repugnant and ethically unjustifiable, and so I stopped eating them. Although at one time I enjoyed those foods, I retrained myself to abjure them. I chose other things to satisfy my hunger. I moved such entities from the category of food I would consume to food I would not consume. Such things could be food for me, but I would rather they not be, so I recategorized them both in my mind and in my life.

I highlight these examples to stress that *what* one eats or not is one's consumptive practice, and this differs from *why* one eats (or not) something. Reasons for maintaining or altering a consumptive practice may shift. For example, some overarching rationales behind my own shift away from eating land animal flesh were financial (I was on a student budget) and ethical (I could not intellectually condone how factory farms treat animals). As time passed, my refusal to eat animal flesh stayed the same, yet my rationales came to include personal health, environmental concerns, and social justice solidarity with the vulnerable, often undocumented workers in rendering plants. Later on I discovered additional reasons to continue my non-meat-eating practices: I found vegetarian fare far easier to share with those I want to welcome into my home, and it arouses less resistance and complications than flesh-centered meals.

My reasons shifted though my practice did not. Conversely, I find my actual consumptive practice often influences my rationales. Whereas I once drank cow's milk without much thought, I have decreased my consumption of it in recent years because I was moved, at times, by the ethical conundrums and environmental degradation inherent in the dairy industry, and at other times by the deleterious effect it had on my gut. In brief, what I consider a food and my actual consumption of it is a constantly shifting, impressionable, and communicative relationship. As my age, circumstances, and education change, I adapt my eating.

In brief, the massive "not us" world can be mapped along three axes: is, could, and should. It includes things we do eat and things we do not eat, things we could eat and things we could not eat (primarily because of personal choice), and things we should eat and things we should not eat. This "should" axis is complicated. Some of us use health as a guide for what we should and should not eat, while others of us defer to religious traditions, and many follow the direction of advocates of certain diets. Regardless, ours is a dynamic relationship with the world-not-us that we eat.

Food—those entities of the world we (can/should/not) eat—is a necessarily ever-changing construct. Food is a constantly renegotiated relationship. As the foodways scholars explain, food is where we work out our identities. Because we must eat and must eat frequently, food is perhaps the most fundamental way we demarcate who we are and why. The eaten, those pieces of the world-not-us that we engulf and fold into ourselves, is precisely where we unfold ourselves the most.

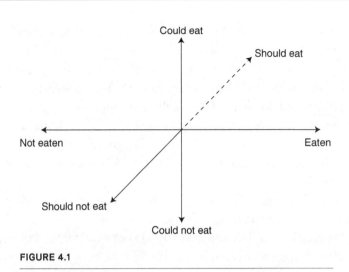

**FIGURE 4.1**

The "not us" world that we eat.

Food is a communicative medium, maybe the most powerful one, through which we convey our understanding of the world, our situation therein, our relationship to it, and our overarching values. What we consider food, what we serve and eat, reveal our convictions.

Consider a highly processed potato chip: What can we say about someone who eats this item? An eater of a highly processed potato chip probably values its taste, convenience, and price. We can further assume about the regular eater of such chips that these values are held more dear than, say, ingredient nutrition and cooking. Were ingredient nutrition truly important to this eater, he or she would opt to eat a real potato instead of its simulation and might even personally cook the potato instead of outsourcing its processing. Circumstances, of course, may constrain an individual's choices, but even within one's situation one's values are reflected in what one chooses to put into one's mouth.

Not all may agree with this claim, of course. According to attested tradition, Jesus contends that what one puts into one's mouth has little to no significance. The eaten neither reflects one's convictions nor impacts one's character. He teaches that "it is not what goes into the mouth that defiles a person, but it is what comes out of the mouth that defiles."[11] Conversely, what one expresses by one's mouth indicates, reflects, and reinforces one's values and commitments. In his view concerns about food misplace energies that should instead be given to one's expressions of faith. One possible reason Jesus advocates this attitude toward food and eating is to distinguish himself and his teachings from the Jewish ways that took the very category of food quite seriously. For Judaism, food and eating most definitely express values and commitments. Thus, for Christianity generally, what food *is* is not a moral category or concern, as it is for many other religious traditions, including Judaism, Islam, Buddhism, and Hinduism.

On the other hand, Jesus maintains that certain foods are indeed morally and even theologically significant. To the masses who were following him through the Gallilee, he preached, "Do not work for food that spoils, but for food that endures to eternal life."[12] As I have already noted, all food is organic, and thus all food must spoil eventually. It cannot be about real, organic food that Jesus speaks, then. He must be referencing some other kind of nourishment. Food here must be a metaphor. He insists that only he can supply this metaphoric food: "I am the bread of life. Your ancestors ate the manna in the wilderness, yet they died. But here is the bread that comes down from heaven, which anyone may eat and not die. I am the living bread that came down from heaven. Whoever eats this bread will live forever. This bread is my flesh, which I will give for the life of the world."[13] Whereas Moses provided organic manna that would eventually spoil to nourish fleshy bodies that would ultimately die and decay, Jesus now offers a radically new kind of food that will enable the consumer to endure eternally.[14] His generosity is undeniable: he freely gives his very body to the collective (believing) body. This special food will not only have wondrous effects on the consumers; it will also convey their beliefs, values, and visions of what the world is and can be. Food—and this food especially—is ethical in and of itself.

Dwell for a moment on the fact that Jesus declares this metaphoric food so symbolically and theologically powerful. Because it is his word that makes this food so special, his is an illocutionary act, a speech whose very utterance transforms reality. Through his words his flesh is no longer *just* flesh; it is *also* food, something in and of the world that can and should be eaten. On his account, his very body is good and laudable food.

How do we know this? Not unlike today's advocates of particular foods and peculiar diets, we have to take Jesus at his word that this food does what he says it does. Epistemologically speaking, we are left to trust Jesus that this food has such capacities; science and experience have yet to corroborate his claims. It could be argued that evidence contradicts his literal claims insofar as no one who has consumed that special food actually lives forever. Such contradictory evidence is not dissimilar to how science continues to demonstrate the dubiousness of the claims of modern diet fads and ads. Yet to be fair, lack of evidence does not mean evidence of lack. Because the possibility for eternal life still remains a possibility, civilization will have to wait to see whether Jesus's claim about this ideal food is indeed true.

## CANNIBALISM

Jesus asserts that there is at least one food that is inherently ethical insofar as the consumption of it articulates one's convictions and identity and would be adaptive in the eternal sense. That singular thing that he encourages us to consider *as a food* is something that hitherto had not been categorized as something of the world that could or should be eaten. Before his declaration making it so, this thing was not human food. Understandable, then, is the confusion subsequent to his declaration:

> Then the Jews began to argue sharply among themselves, "How can this man give us his flesh to eat?" Jesus said to them, "Very truly I tell you, unless you eat the flesh of the Son of Man and drink his blood, you have no life in you. Whoever eats my flesh and drinks my blood has eternal life, and I will raise them up at the last day. For my flesh is real food and my blood is real drink. Whoever eats my flesh and drinks my blood remains in me, and I in them. Just as the living Father sent me and I live because of the Father, so the one who feeds on me will live because of me. This is the bread that came down from heaven. Your ancestors ate manna and died, but whoever feeds on this bread will live forever."[15]

This statement is profound. Jesus no longer speaks about this special food as a metaphor; it is *real* food. And the food about which he speaks is human flesh.

Through another illocutionary act, Jesus hereby recategorizes human flesh from "the uneaten" to "the eaten." Before this teaching, the consumption of human flesh was understood (by Jews, which Jesus was) to be so heinous that it ought not to be considered a possibility at all. Such antipathy toward cannibalism is evident in many biblical passages, including those describing consequences for ignoring or disobeying God and God's instructions.[16] The very idea of consuming human flesh was so repulsive that cannibalism was deployed as a rhetorical strategy to induce compliance. These biblical texts loudly proclaim that the human body is not to be eaten; it is not and should never become food.[17]

Yet an argument can be made that since the Bible repeatedly made these arguments there must have been a need for them. Perhaps there were some people who *did* view cannibalism as both intelligible and healthful. For them, the human body *could* be consumed, even if the act was in some sense reprehensible or human flesh a repugnant source of nourishment. The Bible's consistent antipathy against such cannibalism insists that even if human bodies belong in the section of the world that could be eaten, they should not be eaten.

Jesus disagrees with that initial biblical attitude. For him, the idea of eating human flesh is not inherently evil or depraved, nor should it be a last-resort punishment for waywardness. He flips this logic on its head by saying that consuming human flesh (his, of course, and no one else's) is the very demonstration of acknowledging God and abiding by God's will. On the other hand, Jesus's position could also be the exception proving the rule. *Only* his body may be considered food; *all other* human bodies may never be considered edible. The generic human body must ever remain in the category of the uneaten.

In 1729, the Anglo-Irish satirist Jonathan Swift challenged this logic. In *A Modest Proposal*, Swift advocates the political plausibility and benefits of consuming members of the underclass as a way to address overcrowding, transgenerational poverty, and other social ills. Swift's proposal was satiric precisely because the very idea of consuming conspecifics repulses us. Consider the biblical story about when Ben-Hadad, the king of Aram, besieged Samaria and cut its food supply. Since there was nothing left to eat, one woman killed her own child so she and her neighbor could eat and live another day. When the Samarian king Jehoram learned about this, he became desperately distraught.[18] Consider, too, the famous incident in July 1816 involving the French frigate *Méduse*. After running aground about thirty miles off shore, 150 sailors cast themselves adrift upon a makeshift raft. For a while they resisted the idea and practice of eating fellow humans, who were, admittedly, already dead and still aboard. During the next thirteen days, the calamitous situation did lead many to capitulate to their hunger and engage in anthropophagy.[19] Only fifteen sailors were rescued. Such extreme situations in which cannibalism ultimately occurred demonstrate that even dire circumstances do not necessarily obliterate long-held values, including the values about what one could and should not eat. Our theological and philosophical taboos are strong, but not impervious.

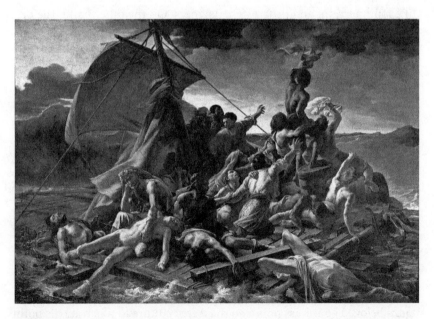

**FIGURE 4.2**

Théodore Géricault, *La Radeau de la Méduse*, 1819.

Biologically, though, when circumstances make human flesh the only source of nutrition available, an argument can be made to consider it food. Human bodies are hardly different, biologically speaking, from the animal bodies we regularly eat. Like those chickens and cows and pigs and sheep and goats and buffalo and deer and fish of many sorts, we too are concatenations of flesh, blood, sinews, bones, skin. Our human bodies also have delicious and nutritious elements—muscle tissue, collagen, elastin, and fat—ready for the taking. Despite the fact that we *could* consider human flesh food, we are not wont to.

Kass identifies several possible reasons for this near universal reticence to think of humans as food. He distinguishes endocannibalism, when the eaten is a member of one's group, from exocannibalism, when the eaten is an outsider or enemy. On his account, the taboo to consider strangers food seems counterintuitive, evolutionarily speaking, because there could be "some selective advantages of eating members of one's own species, provided that one refrains from eating one's own *kin*."[20] Eating nonkin conspecifics is one sure way to get rid of competitors for limited resources like food, terrain, and procreative partners. On the other hand, the origins of the taboo against eating any fellow human, kin or not, may be precisely from intuition itself. Humans naturally and independently discerned that human differences are part of the "promise of human nature," meaning the taboo "is necessary for the perfection of that [diverse] nature."[21] For Kass, "anthropophagy embodies, in principle, a false view of human life . . . [because it] is that extreme of inhumanity regarding eating, more beastly than anything found among the beasts."[22]

Kass's hostility toward cannibalism is both strong and strange. Other humans, especially members of other social groups, are indeed other; they are "not us." Biologically speaking, they are organic members of the world around us theoretically available for our own personal consumption. We *could* eat human flesh, just as we eat chickens, but we typically opt not to. There are some communities and cultures that on occasion eat human flesh in what Kass calls "ritual cannibalism." They eat humans for nonphysiological ends: for revenge or to incorporate, propitiate, or imitate a beloved god. Kass points to the Aztec culture to illustrate his point about endocannibalism: they sacrificed humans to their gods and subsequently ate the bodies.

Yet Kass is strangely silent in regard to Jesus's call to eat his body, now known as the Eucharist. Insofar as only Christians may receive Communion, would this be endo- or exocannibalism? Is it anthropophagy or theophagy, the eating of one's god? How is it more beastly than the beasts? For students of the Eucharist and many of its practitioners, Jesus's fleshy body is hardly beastly but divine, and the consumption of it all the more so. Its transubstantiation—its transformation from a particular human body into ubiquitous wine and bread—offers for the believer real divine nourishment. At one level it may be anthropophagy, at another theophagy, at a third the true expression of one's beliefs and values.[23]

This ambiguity may have informed Protestant discomfort with Roman Catholic literalism of the Eucharist. While the early reformers objected to envisioning the Eucharist wafer and wine as Jesus's actual body, Dositheus, the seventeenth-century leader of Eastern Orthodoxy in Jerusalem, insisted that the Mystery of the sacred Eucharist was true, through and through:

> In the celebration whereof *we believe the Lord Jesus Christ to be present [in the Eucharist]*, not typically, nor figuratively, nor by superabundant grace, as in the other Mysteries, nor by a bare presence, as some of the Fathers have said concerning Baptism, or by impanation [a medieval theory that there is no substantive change in either the bread or Jesus's body], so that the Divinity of the Word is united to the set forth bread of the Eucharist hypostatically, as the followers of Luther most ignorantly and wretchedly suppose. *But [he is present in the Eucharist] truly and really, so that after the consecration of the bread and of the wine, the bread is transmuted, transubstantiated, converted and transformed into the true Body Itself of the Lord*, which was born in Bethlehem of the ever-Virgin, was baptised in the Jordan, suffered, was buried, rose again, was received up, sits at the right hand of the God and Father, and is to come again in the clouds of Heaven; and the wine is converted and transubstantiated into the true Blood Itself of the Lord, Which as He hung upon the Cross, was poured out for the life of the world [as it says in John 6:51].[24]

Dositheus further asserted that in and through consecration, all the bread and wine used at the various churches around the world become and are the true Body and Blood of Jesus. Ultimately, this "Mystery is the greatest, and is spoken of as wonderful, and comprehensible by faith only." For Dositheus and his followers, consuming the Eucharist was nothing less than eating Jesus Christ himself.

The varying levels of agreement and divergence within Christianity about the Eucharist, as well as Kass's aversion to all forms of cannibalism, give voice to an ongoing concern about the ethics of consuming human bodies. They all agree that the human body (or at most, Jesus's body) *can* be consumed; they disagree about whether it should be, by whom, and why.

## CHOICE AND DISGUST

The human body serves to illustrate that even though humans are omnivores, we do not consume everything in the world that we could. Some portions of that edible world we find repugnant, disgusting even. But what is disgust, and how is it related to food and eating?

The word *disgust* is based upon the Latin word for "opposite" or "aversion" (*dis*) and the verb "to taste" (*gustare*). That which our taste would rather avoid we deem disgusting. Curiously, Germanic descendants of *gustare* include *kostan*, which, besides "to taste," means "to choose" and "to cost." That which we find disgusting is often costly to choose.

Disgust is one powerful reason to consider human flesh not food. Like Kass, most people find the very idea of eating fellow humans abhorrent, some kind of perversion of the human eater and the human being eaten, not to mention human nature itself. However depraved and disgusting cannibalism may seem, it nonetheless has a profound if not paradoxical relationship with what is esteemed. Kass rightly points out this dialectical dynamic when he says, "What is held to be disgraceful or disgusting necessarily points to—and is informed by—what is held to be honorable and humanly fine."[25] This holds true for food: some foods we find disgusting precisely because they inversely indicate food we find desirable, admirable, ennobling. I will explore how the tasty and what is tasteful and proper interact in a later chapter.

No less than Charles Darwin, the nineteenth-century naturalist, connected disgust with food and eating, and even class and race. In *The Expression of the Emotions in Man and Animals*, he made this observation:

> The term "disgust," in its simplest sense, means something offensive to the taste. It is curious how readily this feeling is excited by anything unusual in the appearance, odour, or nature of our food. In Tierra del Fuego a native touched with his finger some cold pre-served meat which I was eating at our bivouac, and plainly showed utter disgust at its softness; whilst I felt utter disgust at my food being touched by a naked savage, though his hands did not appear dirty. A smear of soup on a man's beard looks disgusting, though there is of course nothing disgusting in the soup itself. I presume that this follows from the strong association in our minds between the sight of food, however circumstanced, and the idea of eating it.[26]

Darwin makes an important distinction between something *appearing* to be disgusting and something that is *inherently* disgusting or abhorrent to our taste buds. Our eyes and minds play significant roles in our experience of disgust: they mediate between and connect those things that cause us to have a disgusting reaction and our actual response.

Disgust studies—yes, there is such a field—find that disgust is universal: all cultures express it.[27] Disgust is multidimensional, having both immediate and durable features. Its momentary or instantaneous experience includes an affect dimension, a collection of emotional responses that are reflex-like. These are triggered automatically, have a rapid onset, and quickly dissipate. These responses entail signature behavioral, physiological, and attendant qualitative feelings. The automatic behavioral gesture of disgust includes the facial expression of a nose wrinkle, extrusion of the tongue and expelling motion of the mouth, wrinkled upper brow—or what is known as "the gape face." We now associate a simplified depiction of the gape face with poison.

Physiological elements of disgust include a drop in body temperature and a drop in heart rate and increases in salivation and gastrointestinal

**FIGURE 4.3**

The gape face, or Mr. Yuck.

activity. The qualitative feelings include aversion, revulsion, and repulsion, which can vary in intensity and texture. These three elements—behavioral, physiological, and emotional—constitute the disgust affect program. All humans experience disgust affect programs; they are what makes us us.

Many things trigger disgust, of course, not just food. Since disgust triggers elicit reactions within the gastrointestinal system, they necessarily entail some conscious or subconscious notion of oral incorporation, of putting a disgusting thing into one's mouth. Disgusting objects are treated and thought about in certain characteristic ways. They are captivating—even as we try to distance ourselves from them—and are both memorable and difficult to ignore. They are perceived to be unclean, tainted, and impure. Whether they are so in reality is another matter. Such perception of disgusting objects endures longer than the reflexive and instantaneous aversion mentioned earlier. Once marked as disgusting, an object is seen as having the ability to infect other items with its offensiveness. Physical contact, real or imagined, known history of contact, and even close proximity facilitate contamination sensitivity. There is an unusual power asymmetry vis-à-vis the disgusting: it is far easier to pollute the clean and pure than to clean and purify the contaminated. One explanation for our revulsion to certain triggers is called the parasite avoidance theory (PAT) of disgust. According to PAT, things are disgusting because they are, or we imagine them to be, vectors of infectious diseases.[28]

If these are our natural, and often uncomfortable, responses to the disgusting, what triggers them? What do we consider disgusting?

We have many elicitors of disgust reactions. The London Disgust Scale, for example, distinguishes these disgust elicitor categories: food or animal, sex, lesion, atypical appearance, hygiene, fomite (things that are likely to carry infection).[29] In regard to food, disgusting foods should be differentiated from those foods that are inappropriate (e.g., pebbles and chairs—the world-not-us that we cannot and do not eat) and from those that are distasteful because we do not like their taste or imagine we do not like their taste (e.g., *balut*, a Southeast Asian dish with a partially developed duck fetus still in its shell). Of course, no single food will trigger disgust universally. This is a key observation: despite disgust's biological universality, it targets highly idiosyncratic substances. What is disgusting to me may be perfectly acceptable to you, and vice versa.

Consider again the Eucharist. For believers, the wafer and wine are truly Jesus's flesh and blood. His transubstantiation from one edible form into another is in many ways both a profound gesture of hospitality and a significant challenge to human disgust. He chose to become a food that many hold to be disgusting but nonetheless a food they could and would readily take into their own mouths and bodily incorporate. Paradoxically, Jesus taught that though he would be consumed when believers eat his flesh/bread and blood/wine and he would reside within them, they themselves would abide within him.[30] In Jesus's view, what we engulf—even the disgusting—uncovers our own identity. By considering Jesus food and consuming him, we come to exist within him, within the Church, the community of God, the network of the world.

Yet regardless of how much believers may want to consume Jesus, he cannot be devoured completely. This is true both physically and theologically. No single believer or community can consume him so that nothing remains: the Eucharist will be—and must be—offered again. True nourishment from this unique food source comes not from eating one's fill but from eating just enough . . . for now. One is to be satisfied with eating less than one could consume.

In this way disgust, digestion, choice, and identity all interact. The eaten, those pieces of the world-not-us that we take into our mouths, are chosen for myriad reasons. Some we eat because we like them and find them tasty or nutritious physiologically. Some we once ate but no longer do. Some we do not eat because we consider them disgusting. Some we eat despite our real or potential disgust of them. Some we eat because in so doing we convey our identities.

Of the rest of the world we do not eat because eating it would be maladaptive; it would kill us or harm us in some significant way. Vast chunks of the world fall into the category "do not eat." This has not always been a static category, however. In recent centuries, industry and many other social forces have broadened this do-not-eat category so that we eat today far fewer species of plants and animals than did our ancestors. Our modern diet is not less varied, but it is less diverse. We create manufactured foodstuffs the likes of which our ancestors could not have imagined, and many of us have access to cuisines from various parts of the world. By the talents of our own hands we keep our diets interesting, though perhaps if not probably to our distress.

Most of what we eat is a choice. As omnivores, we could eat so much around us but we choose to eat only a portion of the world. To be sure, our choices are often constrained by culture, by economic circumstance, by geological location, and more. Yet what I consider a food is really and ultimately up to me, not someone or something else. I, the eater, am the one eating this particular food. I must eat; no government, company, or religious tradition does or could eat. They may inform, persuade, scare, restrict or inspire me into thinking some edible thing may or may not be eaten. Ultimately, however, I choose whether I put this (disgusting) thing into my mouth, and by doing so I express myself. I need to understand what I consider food, not what others do. I need to understand food from the inside, from *my* inside. I, the eater, eat this world.

# 5

## EATING

*The organism must appear as a function of metabolism rather than metabolism as a function of the organism.*

—Hans Jonas, *The Phenomenon of Life* (1966)

*The Creator, while forcing men to eat in order to live, tempts him to do so with appetite and then rewards him with pleasure.*

—Jean Anthelme Brillat-Savarin, *The Physiology of Taste* (1999)

T hus far I have established that subjects—eaters—take into themselves objects, bits and drips of the world, what I am calling "the eaten." The next question concerns the verb, the very process of taking the world into oneself. What is eating, and why should we care about it?

Some of us may balk here and resist this question's relevance. Since we *must* eat, why question it? Why investigate this act necessary for existence? Some might argue that our mental plates are already full with all the worry about getting food from farm to forks or about complying with a diet. Why should we also worry about the act of moving food from plate to palate, of lifting our forks to our tongues, of chewing and swallowing and digesting and, ultimately, eliminating what we take in?

I could argue that insofar as my eyes cannot see my mouth, which means I am physically blind to my own eating, I may or perhaps even should be mentally ignorant of it as well. Or perhaps I could argue that instead of worrying about my own eating, and since I can easily see others eat, it would be better to talk about your eating or someone else's eating. While I could literally see the activity about which we speak, it would leave me out of the conversation. Indeed, my absence would suggest I have little to no responsibility for my own eating. Such is-to-ought reasoning is specious, however.

I could also shut down the conversation altogether by pointing out that eating predominantly occurs inside the body and thus evades easy observation. Because eating is so hidden, we cannot ascertain with much accuracy or exhaustiveness all that happens inside our mouths or bellies or guts. Uncertainty means that whatever is said about eating is partial at best, and in the worst instances is dangerous. If inaccuracy is the best we can do, why bother talking about eating at all, mine or yours? Such epistemological skepticism would silence most every conversation, though.

Or I could assert that eating is what I do; it is not who I am. So leave my eating alone. However much such defiance may be attractive, it nonetheless betrays the dire need for better appreciation of what eating is and how central it is to our bodily existence. For without eating, without this dynamic relationship with the eaten, every eater will surely die and die sooner than had eating been done. An entity that does not eat cannot rightly be considered an eater at all.

Yet it would be wrong to say that all noneating entities are dead because some may not have been alive in the first place. Rocks, for example, do not die, nor do they live, and they certainly do not eat. *Eating* is a verb of the living. It pertains to organisms existing in dynamic relationship with the world around them. As Kass pithily puts it, "One is only if and because one eats."[1]

While eating is something the living do, it is a relationship of the living with the living, the formerly living, and the nonliving. It is a dynamic interaction between the eater, the world at large, and the eaten in particular. In profound ways, eating bridges the self and the other. It transacts and exchanges. Kass rightfully calls eating transitive: it is done to an other. It mediates, connecting eaters and the eaten and, strangely, the noneaten. Eating also obliterates this very distance by ushering the other's otherness into the self and, eventually and conversely, putting parts of the self out into the world.

Even as eating mediates and connects, it is also immediate: a relation with no middle.[2] Eating is vital for life; lives cannot but eat. Hence the counterintuitive observation by the twentieth-century German and American philosopher of science Hans Jonas: "The organism must appear as a function of metabolism rather than metabolism as a function of the organism."[3] Organisms depend on or are contingent on metabolism; without it, they cannot survive.

Eating matters, then, because it joins my body's matter with the world around me as well as those with whom I (do not) eat, just as it joins your matter with the world around you and those with whom you (do not) eat. Eating thereby and undeniably joins both of us together, even though we may not know each other or live near each other, much less consume (near) each other. My eating implicates your eating, and vice versa. The Australian scholar of gender and cultural studies Elsbeth Probyn reflects on this vibrant relationship: "Rather than simply confirming who we are, eating conjoins us in a network of the edible and inedible, the human and non-human, the animate and the inanimate. In these actions, the individual is constantly connecting, disconnecting and reconnecting with different aspects of individual and social life."[4] Even as Probyn agrees that the eater eating the eaten is an ethically fraught and identity-forming activity, her language of connection reinforces the metaphor of eating as a bridge: eating links, ties, binds, and joins together two distinct entities or parties. However, this rhetoric glosses over a critical feature of eating: along the way, the middle drops out. At some point as eating occurs, no middle, space, or difference exists between the eater and the eaten. The seam dissolves. Eating more than merely connects parts of the world, like self and the world-not-me. It simultaneously brings two together (the eater and the eaten) and destroys their distinctiveness: the eaten becomes deformed and incorporated, literally, into the eater. The other's otherness is obliterated by the self, and whatever energy the other may have had becomes, in part, a part of the self. What eating connects, it absorbs.

In this way eating more than binds us and the world; it blurs this supposed binary. Eating makes it difficult to truly ascertain where I, the eater, start and end and where the world-not-me ends and begins. *Eating* is the verb of profound paradoxes: it dissolves this other into me even as it distinguishes me from all others. Eating *does* so much it's unsurprising that the twentieth-century British anthropologist Mary Douglas calls food "a field of action."[5]

Though many of us may simply eat, eating is no simple activity. In profound ways, eating is miraculous. "To be able to eat and drink," Levinas writes, "is a possibility as extraordinary, as miraculous, as the crossing of the Red Sea. . . . [To] satisfy one's hunger is the marvel of marvels."[6] This, because according to a midrash, each drop of rain that nourished your food was guided by thousands of angels to reach its proper destination. "Nothing is as difficult as being able to feed oneself!"[7] Levinas proclaims. This difficult, necessary, even miraculous daily act needs our attention.

To better understand this complicated activity called eating, I will begin by exploring what Plato, Aristotle, and Spinoza have to say, because, as noted earlier, they have shaped how we think about our relation with food and eating itself. Then I will look at our primary appetites, homeostasis, the drive to replenish our energy, and hedonism, the drive to enjoy. Such appetites are incessant and require constant attention and physical effort. This effort is metabolism, which includes ingestion, digestion, and egestion, among other activities. Further reflections on eating unveil more of its paradoxical features and lead us to the central question of this whole project: What does it mean to eat well?

## APPETITES

What drives eating? Whence the urge to take the world-not-us into ourselves to taste its juices and absorb its energies? Such questions have an ancient lineage. For thousands of years, students of the human condition meditated on our drive to eat, and they gave it a name: *appetite.*

Plato teaches that appetite and sexual drives intermingle. They are managed in that part of the soul situated in the lower midriff just above the navel. He identifies two other parts of the soul: the spirited one, housed in the heart, that manages anger and courage, and the rational one, humming in the mind. Only the rational part is immortal; the other two die with the mortal body. Ideally, the rational part governs the other two. Though the appetites may be the lowest part of this tripartite soul, their import is significant and location purposive:

> And all that part of the Soul which is subject to appetites for foods and drinks, and all the other wants that are due to the nature of the body, they are planted in the parts midway between the midriff and the boundary at the navel, fashioning as it were a manger in all this region for the

feeding of the body; and there they tied up this part of the Soul, as though it were a creature which, though savage, they must necessarily keep joined to the rest and feed, if the mortal stock were to exist at all. In order, then, that this part, feeding thus at its manger and housed as far away as possible from the counselling part, and creating the least possible turmoil and din, should allow the Supreme part to take counsel in peace concerning what benefits all, both individually and in the mass [that is, the whole body], for these reasons they [the gods fashioning the human body] stationed it in that position.[8]

To put Plato in modern terms: though the immortal rational mind must be chained to this lowly savage beast—the bodily soul dealing with hunger and sex—slurping at its trough, the physical distance between them buffers the physique's clamor below so that reason can hear itself and make decisions for the whole organism's benefit.

Appetite, for Plato, is simultaneously unruly and indispensable for human existence. It can be and is meant to be controlled by the rational and reasoning mind. On the other hand, Plato's view of appetite acknowledges the possibility that it can run amok. Its wild hungers and impulses could overpower the mind, and the mind, biologically chained to the body, is dragged along for the ride.

About a century later, Aristotle takes a slightly different tack. He distinguishes two kinds of appetite: those that are natural and common across all creatures and those that are peculiar to individuals and are acquired. The urge to eat and drink is a natural and generic drive all sentient beings share, human and nonhuman alike. By contrast, preferences for particular kinds of food or drink are peculiar to each individual. In his words, "different things are pleasant to different kinds of people, and some things are more pleasant to everyone than chance objects."[9] Certainly we often enjoy eating food, and yet there are some foods we particularly enjoy eating. Bodily sustenance and alimentary enjoyment are thus two distinct kinds of appetite. In today's terms, these are the homeostatic and hedonistic drives.

Enjoyment or pleasure is not uniform, of course. Nor is enjoyment the ultimate good; it is *a* good, one among many.[10] For Aristotle, the question is not whether one enjoys what one is doing but whether it ennobles, whether it is virtuous in and of itself. An activity's virtue matters more than the enjoyment one experiences from it. Since enjoyment is merely derivative or secondary, pleasure or hedonism cannot be one's ultimate goal. As actions should aim to be virtuous, in the case of eating, the virtue that should shape one's eating ought to be temperance, a practice I will discuss in a later chapter. The mind thus needs to wrest control of the appetite to inculcate such good behavior.

About two thousand years later, in the seventeenth century, Spinoza agrees that appetite is necessary for the very existence and preservation of each individual. And like Aristotle, he thinks the mind is capable of controlling appetites. But Spinoza adds another ingredient to the mix: consciousness. Being conscious of one's appetite is central to his definition of desire. Though all animals have appetites, or bodily strivings, only humans are conscious of those strivings; only humans desire per se. "From all this," Spinoza claims, "it is clear that we neither strive for, nor will, neither want, nor desire, anything because we judge it to be good; on the contrary, we judge something to be good because we strive for it, will it, want it, and desire it."[11]

Spinoza hereby reframes the famous question posed many millennia earlier by Socrates to Euthyphro: "Is the holy loved by the gods because it is holy, or is it holy because it is loved by the gods?"[12] Either way, the object (be it the holy or the good) is valued positively because it already is that quality or is that quality precisely because we (or the gods) consider it so. For Socrates, an object is loved precisely because of its innate qualities: the gods love the holy because it is holy. Whether they love it is inconsequential to its holiness. This raises a strange category at the edges of theological and philosophical ethics of objects that are simultaneously holy and unloved.

Still, for Spinoza, an object is deemed good not because there is something about or in it for which we yearn. It is our striving, desiring, wanting, and willing a thing that makes it good. Insofar as these impulses are innate and automatic, our cognitive evaluation or judgment of the object is secondary. Judgment's tardiness suggests we cannot rightfully rely upon it as a guide for our actions. This is especially true when it comes to such existential choices regarding our very nourishment. Cognitive assessment is already too late. We would do better to rely upon our preconscious impulses: we should rely upon our appetites.

Spinoza thus calls for our conscious mind to be ever more aware of our preconscious drives. The more we are aware, the more adequate our ideas will be about what we do, why, and how. The more we know about what we do, why, and how, the more we become like God—who, obviously, knows everything. Insofar as we are material beings, we can *never* be God, who is immaterial. However, Spinoza is more concerned about our becoming better human beings, not divine beings. The more knowledge we have of our hidden desires and impulses, the more control we can exercise over them. Paradoxically, then, the more we know about our bodies and their appetites, the more control we can have of our bodily selves and the more freedom we can experience.

Philosophically speaking, appetite is an inevitable, ineradicable feature of creaturely existence. Humans are no exception: we are appetitive organisms. As an endogenous drive, appetite motivates us to be ever outwardly oriented, always looking for that which is not-us that could satisfy bodily needs and please our palates. If left unchecked or intellectually abandoned because so hidden, appetite could bring about maladaptive eating strategies that would endanger the organism itself. Another paradox of eating is that, left to its own devices, appetite could eat itself to death. Appetite known and managed, by contrast, could engender adaptive, healthy—even virtuous—eating strategies.

Contemporary studies of appetite corroborate such philosophical reflections.[13] They distinguish two kinds of appetites: hedonism and homeostasis. These two appetites drive human consumption. The more we can understand them, the better our chances are to develop, practice, and embrace eating strategies healthy for our particular bodies.

I once heard someone say that humans are eating tubes surrounded by flesh. We are more complicated than that, of course, but our very organism ensures its own viability and vitality, and this continuous effort requires energy that itself must be extracted from the more-than-us world, which is food. This kind of drive or appetite to ensure an organism's existence can be called homeostatic.

Homeostasis is the appetite that seeks to replenish an organism's energy. *Homeo*, Greek for "self," and *stasis* or "status": a system that regulates itself at a fairly stable rate. The very idea of homeostasis came not from a study of the human body and its appetites but from the movement of fluid between cells. A nineteenth-century French physiologist, Claude Bernard, called the constant equilibration of fluids and pressures between and within cells *milieu intérieur*, or "interior milieu," and it is this "stability of the internal environment [that] is the condition for the free and independent life."[14]

An organic system can survive and even thrive by ensuring a stable internal environment. Brillat-Savarin a few years before Bernard hinted at this idea in his animated study of human existence and eating: "Movement and life cause a steady loss of substance in any living being; and the human body, that highly complicated machine, would soon be useless if Providence had not placed in it a sentinel which sounds a warning the moment its resources are no longer in perfect balance with its needs. This guardian is appetite, by which is meant the first warning of the need to eat."[15] The sentinel appetite that seeks to maintain the internal balance, a steady state of "substance" or energy, is the homeostatic appetite.

Though the idea of systemwide equilibrium may have made its rounds in mid-nineteenth-century France, the term *homeostasis* would be coined by Walter Bradford Cannon at Harvard in his 1932 *Wisdom of the Human Body* to explain why blood temperature and sugar levels were continuously maintained. Cannon connected the term to appetite: "Thirst, as well as hunger, may be explained as means of providing the supplies needed for homeostasis in the internal environment."[16] Thirst and hunger, then, are essential components of the body's homeostatic system. They signal the organism to consume exogenous foodstuffs and thus bring into itself additional energy. From Cannon's influence, this drive to regain bodily energy supplies would be called the homeostatic appetite.

To be sure, the mechanisms constituting the homeostatic appetite are many. Research now shows that appetite is more complex than an empty or emptying stomach conveying its spatial lack to give the brain a cue for the body to seek and consume food and drink. Both positive and negative feedback loops result. The positive loop involves the food itself. Its smells, sounds, and sights encourage consumption, as does its temperature, texture, and taste once it is in the mouth. Such stimuli encourage eating. Once the food has reached the stomach, however, its role changes.

This ingested food begins to fill the belly, and this volumetric distension signals to the brain that the belly can contain only so much more. Once food leaves the mouth, it thus becomes a part of the negative feedback loop to slow and stop eating. Digested foods—both that which remains in the stomach and that which leaves it for the duodenum, small intestine, and beyond—are part of the negative feedback loop.

I will say more momentarily about digestion; for now it should be noted that even when homeostatic appetite runs smoothly, it is nonetheless influenced by myriad other stimuli. External pressures on the body may be the environment in which food is being consumed, the social setting, and the like. Internal pressures also influence consumption: stress, maladies, and so on. Hormones, too, play a significant role in eating.

Because hormones are so critical to homeostatic eating, modulating eating from beginning to evacuation, it can be said that "the gastrointestinal tract is the largest endocrine organ of the body."[17] The major hormones include glucagon-like peptide (GLP)-1, peptide YY (PYY), pancreatic polypeptide (PP), oxyntomodulin (OXM), and ghrelin. Except for ghrelin, all are anorexigenic: they suppress eating; because it stimulates eating, ghrelin is orexigenic. The anorexigenic hormones, secreted by sections of the gastrointestinal tract below the stomach, signal to the brain when adequate nutrition has been transferred to and through it. These hormones eventually squelch appetite, which in turn shuts off eating. Conversely, ghrelin signals hunger to the brain. Its powerful neuronal stimulus combines with physical sensations of lack in the stomach (from mechanoreceptors) to produce a powerful impetus to consume. Unlike the suppressive hormones, ghrelin is secreted by the stomach itself.

Altogether these hormones create a positive and negative feedback loop between gut and brain. As mentioned in chapter 2, this loop is a sophisticated mechanism that protects the organism from both starvation and hyperphagia (overeating) if it operates unimpeded and is heeded. It facilitates adaptive eating strategies.

Some scientists contend that manipulating the anorexigenic hormones could efficiently and effectively regulate eating, especially obesigenic eating. They hold that "it therefore seems not unreasonable to propose that in the therapeutic targeting of appetite regulation, polypharmacy with a number of therapies might maximize clinical effect while minimizing side effects, mirroring trends in the management of other chronic conditions such as hypertension."[18] Put in other terms, this proposal would have people use many pills that interfere with their gastrointestinal hormones to regulate maladaptive eating patterns.

Other scientists disagree with this reactive and rather medicalized suggestion. For them, reliance upon hormones to communicate "stop" to the brain is too late and too weak. It takes twenty-plus minutes for eating-suppressing hormones to convey messages to the brain to stop eating. Much can be consumed in those twenty minutes. In fact, those twenty minutes could very well be the deadliest in our lives, for during them we ingest more than our bodies need. Another reason hormones may not be the best mechanism for regulating one's eating is that they are so subtle. Paying attention to them is difficult, if not impossible. Attuning oneself to one's hormonal fluctuations requires not only incredible self-awareness but such awareness that can override extremely distracting external cues and influences. Even the advocates of the pharmacological intervention admit that their proposal is incomplete: "The development of an effective gut hormone-based therapy will not absolve patients from the responsibility for their own lifestyle."[19] Hormone pills alone will not suffice.

As our judging minds are too late to regulate our eating and our hormones are both too late and too weak, a better way to control our eating looks to physical sensations. Before we get to what those are, let's follow food as it enters our bodies.

Our mouths open for the stuff of the world-not-us that we elect to put into our bodies. Once it is there, our teeth set to work masticating—chewing, ripping, shredding, chomping, mashing—and our salivary glands add protease (protein digester) and lipase (fat digester) to aid digestion farther down the tract. The tongue swishes food and saliva together into clumps called boluses, pushes these to the back of the mouth, and then swallows them.

As amazing as it is that our teeth and jaws are so powerful, that our jaws do not destroy our own teeth is perhaps even more incredible. We chew hard when needed, but not so hard as to harm ourselves. Something in our subconscious brains stops our jaws from smashing our own teeth to bits. The nineteenth-century American dentist Greene Vardiman Black discovered with his gnathodynamometer that our jaws create incredible force when biting and chewing, yet we do not shatter our own teeth.[20] Such self-protective mechanisms exist throughout the alimentary canal. For example, the stomach's acids dissolve most everything they touch, but not the stomach itself. The intestinal villi absorb nutrients from passing food and refrain from absorbing each other. Such facts prove that our alimentary canals from beginning to end are designed to consume the world-not-us.

After being swallowed, a bolus travels down the esophagus and passes into the churning stomach. Each swallow sends more volume of food and drink into the stomach, which continues to expand to accommodate the new arrivals. This physical distension of the stomach is immediate. Not unlike a balloon, the stomach expands to a normal volume at which it is neither overblown nor underinflated. Until that point, its mechanoreceptors send signals to the brain that the stomach has not yet reached optimal size; it seeks more. As Brillat-Savarin says, "Appetite declares itself by a vague languor in one's stomach and a slight feeling of fatigue."[21]

But once the stomach has reached its optimal size, eating should stop, for after this stage, each subsequent bolus dropped into the stomach extends and expands it. When stretched beyond normal, the stomach has to work even harder to mechanically massage its contents. We feel uncomfortable after glutting ourselves because we have forced our stomachs into difficult and unnecessary labor.

Extra food is unnecessary, too. When the stomach is filled to its normal capacity, the caloric makeup of the contents is typically adequate for our bodily needs. Anything put into the stomach after that point is superfluous. Study after study shows that those extra calories are literally killing us. Eating beyond that moment of adequacy is deadly.

Eating adequately, or eating enough, can be easily achieved by attending to the physical sensation of our stomach's expansion during a meal. Instead of relying upon hormones that are both subtle and late or upon our delayed judging minds, reacting to our stomach's immediate physical sensations of adequacy promises to be a better and stronger mechanism to promote, regulate, and cease consumption.

The story of eating does not stop with the stomach, of course. As Pavlov famously said, "The physiologist who succeeds in penetrating deeper and deeper into the digestive canal becomes convinced that it consists of a number of chemical laboratories equipped with various mechanical devices."[22] These laboratories plumb ever deeper into the human torso, well beyond the stomach—fascinating as that lab may be.

Food continues down the gastrointestinal tract beyond the stomach's drain stopper, or pyloric sphincter, and into the small intestine, large intestine, colon, and beyond. The rate food empties out of the stomach depends on its volume and energy content, or density. The higher the energy content, the slower food will move beyond the stomach, because the food needs to be broken down into smaller, digestible components. The stomach's hydrochloric acid, gastric acid, pepsin, and other digestive enzymes work chemically in conjunction with the mechanical massaging of the stomach muscles to break the food apart, a process called *catabolism*. The reverse process, *anabolism*, occurs when the body processes the nutrients to build on its cells' components.

One of the things Pavlov discovered in the late nineteenth century is that even food introduced directly into the stomach, bypassing the mouth, with its saliva and taste-, texture-, and temperature-identifying sensitivities, stimulates certain kinds of stomach secretions that are peculiarly geared to catabolize that food. Food, then, acts on the digestive system itself; it is not merely subject to the organism's mechanical and chemical assault. From the mouth to the stomach and beyond, the food put into the alimentary canal chemically communicates to and thus influences the body into which it will eventually be absorbed. Once the food has been adequately disassembled into chyme, the stomach releases it into the duodenum, the topmost part of the small intestine.

Chyme causes the duodenum to secrete cholecystokinin (CKK), a hormone that stimulates the gall bladder to release bile and other digestive enzymes from the pancreas. These chemicals moderate the acidity of the chyme so that the jejunum section of the small intestine can get to work extracting useful nutrients from the passing organic material, which is now called chyle. Lining the walls of the jejunum are millions of villi, small finger-like appendages that themselves have tiny microvilli, all of which absorb the chyle's sugars, amino acids, fats, and vitamins. (The modern word *jejune*, which means "devoid of substance" or "naïve," derives

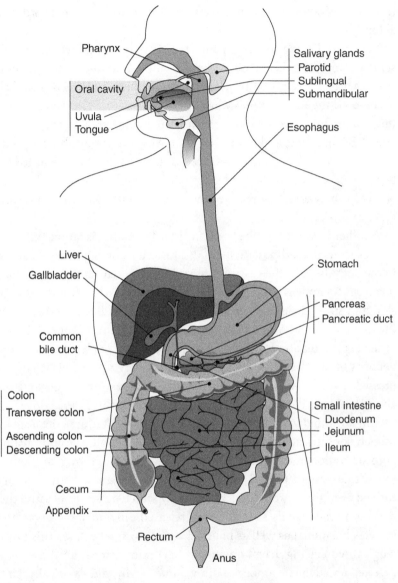

**FIGURE 5.1**

The human digestive system. Courtesy of *Wikipedia*, http://upload.wikimedia.org /wikipedia/commons/c/c5/Digestive_system_diagram_en.svg.

from this section of the gut because it was frequently found empty during autopsies.)

Remaining chyle moves on into the large intestine, which absorbs short-chain fatty acids (SCFA), minerals, and vitamins. Water and electrolytes are also removed from the chyle here. Flora or microbiota help decompose the material into what will become feces. The value of these microbiotic interlopers cannot be overstated. They create such vitamins as B12, K, thiamine, and riboflavin, all of which the body absorbs in this section of the alimentary tract. Once this material has been digested (albeit imperfectly), it is then compacted and stored as stools in the colon and rectum, ready to be released by the anus. Table 5.1 provides a summary of this process.

Another influence on the brain in regard to eating is fat mass. Recent studies show that adipose tissues (also known as fat deposits) elsewhere in the body, beyond the gastrointestinal tract, secrete leptin, another anorexigenic or appetite-suppressing hormone. In theory, leptin should help slow and stop eating. However, "large amounts of adipose tissue, resulting in high circulating levels of leptin, lead to leptin resistance and a lack of the expected anorectic effect."[23] Thus for some people who have large deposits of fat, the naturally suppressive potency of leptin is itself suppressed. Fat's faded signal to stop eating allows eating to continue unabated and thus contribute to even more fatty deposits in the body.[24]

This admittedly brief review shows that homeostatic appetite is an extremely sophisticated feedback mechanism that defends the body against both starvation and overconsumption. Having evolved over millions of years, this system proved adaptive for organisms. They survived and thrived even in environments of relatively scarce nutrition because they had hormonal signals to *stop* eating released only *after* the organ that secretes hormonal as well as physical signals to *start* eating. This physiological sequencing drives organisms to continue to eat until they have ingested an adequate amount both volumetrically and calorically. Until then, the body is designed to continue to eat.

Up to recent centuries, the typical foodstuffs humans consumed were nutritiously basic. Eating until one's stomach was adequately full was a reasonable or adaptive way to maintain a relatively healthy body weight. Today, however, the food environment is dramatically different. In gen-

## TABLE 5.1  WHAT THE BODY DOES TO FOOD

| Organic material | Verb / Noun | Body Part | Process | Additives | Hormones |
|---|---|---|---|---|---|
| Food | Ingest | Mouth | Masticate | Saliva (protease, lipase) | |
| Bolus | Post-ingestion | Esophagus | Transport | | |
| Chyme | Digest | Stomach | Mechanical and chemical mixing | Gastric acid, pepsin, hydrochloric acid | Ghrelin |
| Chyle | Digest | Small intestine | Absorption (vitamins, nutrients, proteins) | | PP, PYY, GLP-1, CCK, OXM |
| Chyle | Digest | Large intestine | Absorption (SCFA, minerals, B, K, $H_2O$, salt) | Microbiota | |
| Feces | Post-digestion | Colon | Hold | | |
| Feces | Egest | Anus | Evacuate | | |

eral terms, food today is superabundant, and much of that food is hyper-palatable. It is no longer basic but manipulated, carefully concocted combinations of salts, sugars, and fats, and it is extremely caloric- and energy-dense. Though consuming such delicious fare may be enjoyable for our mouths and minds, it is something our bodies can barely deal with because they are not yet designed to handle such intense mixtures. Nor are our bodies able to process the influx of calories or proteins. Our homeostatic hormonal system, in brief, is of little and belated help in the contemporary food environment.

Further, since for millennia our bodies only rarely consumed salts, sugars, and fats, our brains are acutely aware when they are present in our foods. Great neurological activity occurs when we ingest such ingredients, and we experience enjoyment. They please us.

Let us turn now to another kind of appetite, the appetite for pleasure. Brillat-Savarin observed that two kinds of appetite operate within us: "At the same time one's soul concerns itself with things connected with its own needs; memory recalls dishes that have pleased the taste; imagination pretends to see them; there is something dreamlike about the whole process. This state is not without its charms, and a thousand times we have heard its devotees exclaim with a full heart: 'How wonderful to have a good appetite, when we are sure of enjoying an excellent dinner before long!' "[25] In short, the body's drive for self-maintenance occurs simultaneously with the desire to enjoy pleasurable dishes. Brillat-Savarin sharpens their difference by adding, "The pleasure of eating is a peculiar sensation directed to the satisfaction of a necessity. The pleasures of the table are a reflected sensation, originating in various facts, places, things and persons."[26] Whereas humans share with animals the pleasure of eating—that is, homeostatic appetite—the other is unique to humans. Only we know the pleasures of the table. They are most evident at our celebrations, when we carefully prepare meals, think about how we serve them, and assemble select fellow eaters. This latter appetite is associated with the social body, the context in which food is consumed. It is also contingent or dependent upon where and when one lives. The other appetite that hungers for self-maintenance is internal to each individual body and is universal across all animals.

Nearly a hundred years later, in 1932, Cannon similarly speaks of two kinds of hunger. In his account, the need to replenish energy stores is the motivator

> for the taking of food and water. Fundamentally these are the disagreeable experiences of hunger and thirst: the unpleasant pangs, which disappear when food is eaten, and the unpleasant dryness of the mouth, which disappears when water or watery drink is drunk. But these automatic "drives" lead at times to delectable sensations of taste and smell. Such sensations become associated with the taking of the special foods and drinks which have occasioned them. Thus appetites are established which, by inviting to eat and to drink, may replace in part the need for the goads of hunger and thirst. But if appetite fails to keep up the supplies, the more imperious and more insistent agencies come into action and demand that the reserves be replenished.[27]

Like Brillat-Savarin, Cannon identifies two appetites operating at the same time. One occurs subconsciously as an automatic drive to diminish the discomforts of hunger and thirst. The other is more conscious insofar as it cognitively associates taste and smell (which are physiologically bound up with each other) of certain foodstuffs with the occasions in which they are ingested. While the latter appetite can supersede the former, the former retains the potential to override the latter should the body's energy be so depleted. This echoes what we saw earlier about hormones: the body is supremely well designed to protect itself from egregious deprivation and starvation.

Both Brillat-Savarin and Cannon thus distinguish the homeostatic appetite, driven to replenish energy stores, from the hedonic appetite, yearning to enjoy delectables. The two appetites are not mutually exclusive, however. While homeostatic appetite stimulates eating to satisfy metabolic needs, we frequently like or want the food that our homeostatic appetite hankers after. Recent studies of the neurobiology of eating find that in the modern world "of abundant palatable foods and food cues,

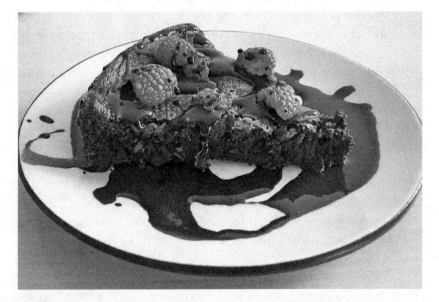

**FIGURE 5.2**

Want some? External cues frequently prompt eating beyond homeostatic replenishment.

brain reward systems of 'liking' and 'wanting' are often activated in the absence of metabolic need."[28] This means that being exposed even to pictures of hyperpalatable foods—as we are in the U.S. food-advertising environment—can trigger more than homeostatic consumption; such cues can prompt maladaptive eating.

Because the very sight of tasty foods can override the innate signal that our metabolic needs have already been met, eating at sumptuous banquets or buffets or even having extra food on the plate and table around us—all these external cues can induce eating beyond what our bodies need. Consider the common phrase "Your eyes are larger than your stomach." It could refer to the habit of ordering too much food at restaurants or of not consuming all the food one puts on one's plate. Both interpretations convey a lack of awareness of how much food one *can* eat. But at a more profound level, the phrase can also refer to how much food one *should* eat. Though our eyes see (or our nose smells) food, consuming it may not be wise; in fact, it could be outright dangerous. Our eyes distract us because they point our attention to external cues. Eating well, by contrast, requires orienting ourselves to internal cues instead.

We should also distinguish liking a food from wanting a food. The set of foods from which we derive pleasure do not remain static in our lives. Rather, even though our brains are highly sensitive to salts, sweets, and fats, most foods start out neutral to our brains. As we experience certain foods over time, our brains form associations between those foods and our enjoyment of them. In time, we come to *like* certain foods. *Wanting* a food is slightly different. Whereas we may like, say, sushi and may not eat it for quite some time, wanting a food is more immediate and urgent. The smell of a freshly baked pie, for example, can "acquire motivational power" in our neurocircuitry and induce eating beyond metabolic needs.[29] Of course, we often like and want a particular food at the same time. But wanting a particular food can motivate us to eat beyond what we like. The statement "I like sushi, but I want this pie right now" thus makes sense.

Just as exposure to certain foods can train our brains to like and want them, hunger also influences the enjoyment we derive from them. Alliesthesia, the phenomenon of liking a particular food, is enhanced when hungry. Similarly, wanting a food is more intense when hungry. Hormonally speaking, studies show that increased ghrelin heightens the incentive properties of certain foods, so when we are hungry our desire for those foods intensifies, which can lead us to consume them beyond our homeostatic needs.[30] When hungry, we would consume more pie (that ingeniously combines salt, sugar, and fats) than our bodies actually need.

What is so important in such studies of hedonic appetite is that we learn what and how to enjoy food. Our societies teach us through exposure and experience to link certain food tastes, sights, and smells with certain kinds of pleasures. Recall your traditional Thanksgiving feast or the annual community pancake breakfast on the Fourth of July, or the collards at the family picnic. Our brains remember such associations, and subsequent eating experiences reinforce them. So, for example, when we have a piece of chocolate cake at our own birthday party, we come to link the happiness of that moment with the taste of the cake. Our brains connect those emotions and sensations, and because they were so positive, we will both like cake and, in some situations, want it too.

Here is the crucial point: just as we can train ourselves to like and want certain foods, we can also train our brains to unlike and not want certain foods.

Hunger can play a powerful role here, if we let it. We can use our hunger to stimulate our desire for certain foods, especially for healthier ones. As we consume those healthier foods, we can link the positive sensations of becoming sated to those healthier foods, thereby creating a positive feedback loop. In this way, we can adjust our hedonic appetites away from unhealthy foods and maladaptive eating practices and toward healthier foods and adaptive eating practices. By turning our gaze away from the bombardment of external cues trying to manipulate our likes and wants in order to pay more attention to our internal cues, we can become more mindful consumers, increasingly aware of "the body's innate physiology to guide eating behaviors."[31]

The idea that we can train our appetites is not new, of course. Pavlov made famous the notion of conditioned reflexes. He found that when exposed to certain stimuli, animals develop certain reactions or reflexes. Take away these direct stimuli and show only the original source to the animal, and those same reflexes appear. For example, Pavlov fed a dog some meat and noted its salivary secretions. He did this repeatedly, imprinting on the dog's mind the association of the meat and its consumption. He then merely showed the dog some meat and observed it drool at the same rate as if it were also eating it. Pavlov also found that repeated exposure to stimuli without the actual engagement eventually dilutes the potency of that reflex; in some cases, the reflex dissolves altogether. A dog shown food it cannot eat will, after some time, no longer salivate.

At least in regard to conditioned reflexes, humans hardly differ from the dogs of Pavlov's experiments. We too will salivate when given food, and after some time will salivate when only shown that food. Many of us will drool with anticipation when our eyes observe hyperpalatable food, like that picture of chocolate pie, or when our nose smells freshly cooked meat. Such reactions mean that we can recondition what we like and want; we need not be slaves to our hedonic appetites.

Our modern economy and culture play on the fact that our appetites are so malleable and impressionable. Businesses find it lucrative to stimulate our minds through ads, since merely seeing a picture of foods and drinks on a screen or page or billboard will get our alimentary juices flowing and our hormones raging. These ads disrupt our attention from whatever it was we were doing, and we begin to look for that particular food or drink because our body is now expecting it, even ready for it. In such stimulated states, we frequently open our wallets and our mouths to consume things that bring us the briefest moment's enjoyment. No wonder Kass laments that those who eat for a "timeless and purposeless hedonic present . . . disseminate the evils that come from mistaking the pleasant for the good."[32]

Yet, hedonic eaters do not consume only those foods that please them. Indeed, people usually eat less of the foods they enjoy most. For example, though an individual may derive more pleasure from chocolate cake than a carrot, it is highly likely that, overall, he or she eats more carrots than chocolate cake.[33]

## EATING IS SUCH A WASTE

Eating, however essential and enjoyable, is not the central verb of life. As Brillat-Savarin pithily observes, *"A man does not live on what he eats,* an old proverb says, *but on what he digests*. It follows then that it is necessary to digest in order to live."[34] Digestion, or absorption, of foodstuffs into the body is not just what enables us to live; digestion is life living.

Digestion is an imperfect activity, however. When Jonas argues that metabolism is an organism's "exchange of matter with the surroundings,"[35] he includes not just the *ingestion* of the world-not-us that we put into our bodies. Metabolism's exchange also includes the matter our bodies *egest*, or eject: our waste.

Rabbi Bahya once wrote, "The nature of eating is the annihilation of the thing that is eaten and made into waste."[36] Not all that we put into our bodies stays there. While some is digested and absorbed into us—and becomes us—much is not. It passes along the alimentary canal, through the small and large intestines, waits for a while in the colon, and eventually passes out through the rectum.

We have long suspected there is a direct correlation between input and output, between what we consume and our feces. Plato in his *Gorgias* reports Socrates's question, "If there's a lot of stuff pouring in, there has to be a lot of stuff leaving as well, doesn't there?"[37] An early medieval rabbinic midrash similarly insists, "One who increases eating increases what is released."[38] Likewise, the Venetian physiologist Santorio Santorii (aka Sanctorius, 1561–1636), the first person to study metabolism scientifically, offered this aphorism in his 1614 *Medicina Statica*: "The natural discharges are not in proportion to the weight of the body, but the quantity of diet taken in."[39]

Sanctorius was fascinated with waste. For thirty years he measured himself regularly on a chair hooked up to a scale; he also measured what he ate and drank and, of course, what he excreted. To his surprise, he found a discrepancy between those numbers: what came out did not equal what went in. He called this discrepancy *perspiratio insensibilis*, "insensible perspiration." Though he linked this insensible perspiration to the skin's pores or the lung's humidity, his idea was quite prescient: recent studies have discerned that our bodies lose about 60 percent of our energy through the heat we produce. The vast majority of this dissipated energy comes from the food we consume. The waste our bodies produce may still contain energy. Not all possible nutrients have been absorbed by our digestive tracts. Fecal matter contains palatable nutrition; indeed,

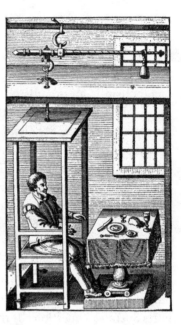

**FIGURE 5.3**

Sanctorius watched his intake and output
for thirty years. From Sanctorius 1720:
frontmatter.

that nutrition is often easier to digest since it has already gone through
the system beforehand (think seeds). Though uncommon, some animals
consume their own waste. Called coprophagy, this behavior is also known
to exist among humans; even the Bible mentions it.[40]

Eating is inherently wasteful because digestion is incomplete. Eating
more than our bodies need or eating until we are full or glutted is all the
more wasteful. These eating strategies all but force our bodies to absorb
energy and nutrients unnecessary for basic metabolic needs. Such excessive consumption also sweeps through our bodies and into sewer systems foodstuffs that could have met metabolic needs of others who are
hungry.

Our appetites and eating have profound impacts on our own bodies
and others'. As Probyn observes, "We are alimentary assemblages, bodies that eat with vigorous class, ethnic and gendered appetites, mouth machines that ingest and regurgitate, articulating what we are, what we eat
and what eats us . . . . [E]ating refracts who we are."[41] It thus behooves us
to think carefully about our eating. We should wonder whether our eating is excessively wasteful, that is, bad. We should also wonder how our
eating could be good or at least better.

Without being hyperbolic, such questions about eating may be *the* issue for humankind. According to the twentieth-century French philosopher Jacques Derrida, these questions about eating dissolve into just one: "The moral question is thus not, nor has it ever been: should one eat or not eat, eat this and not that, the living or the nonliving, man or animal, but since *one must* eat in any case and since it is and tastes good to eat, and since there's no other definition of the good, how for goodness sake should one *eat well*?"[42] For Derrida, our ultimate concern should not be about whether "it is 'good' to eat the other or if the other is 'good' to eat."[43] We should not worry so much about eating per se or eating a specific item. The former is essential for existence, and the latter depends on whom you ask because climate, culture, and class all influence whether a particular eaten thing is considered good. Rather, and most emphatically, the question is *How should one eat well?* While eating well certainly concerns physical features of consumption, eating well is also a moral, even metaphysical activity.

# EATING WELL

*The discovery of a new dish confers more happiness on humanity,
than the discovery of a new star.*

—Jean Anthelme Brillat-Savarin, *The Physiology of Taste* (1999)

# 6

# EATING'S GENESIS

*The morality of "earthly nourishments" is the first morality, the first abnegation. It is not the last, but one must pass through it.*

—Emmanuel Levinas, *Time and the Other* (1987)

At birth, a human baby, if given the opportunity, naturally wiggles its way to its mother's breast to feed. Despite its limited eyesight, a newborn can discern the areola, locate the nipple, and situate it into its mouth and begin to suck. Universally, after taking a breath, the first activity a human does is take from the world around it and consume.[1] Eating is our primordial pursuit. Should we be frustrated, should we not reach or find or grasp that natural source of nourishment, we often burst into wails and squeals. When not given the opportunity to eat or if that first eating opportunity is compromised because of a bad latch or if colostrum does not readily flow, somehow, intuitively, we know something is wrong—and we communicate in the only way we know how: we cry.

Eating is simultaneously our first physical pursuit and our first metaphysical encounter with flourishing. Levinas thus calls eating the first morality, our primordial relation with goodness and what is contrary to goodness. He astutely observes that eating is not our only or last moral conundrum. All others—all other ethically fraught scenarios—are subsequent to this one, our first and incessant need to eat. All those other concerns about which we spend a great deal of energy and resources are concerns precisely because we eat and have already eaten.

That eating is and must be the first concern of a living creature—especially humans—is reflected and reinforced by many religious traditions that situate eating as the first morally significant activity of human existence. No less than the Bible, the foundational text for Judaism and Christianity and to some extent for Islam, describes eating as a primary feature of humankind's genesis. To be sure, the Bible is not, nor does it understand itself to be, a scientific book of biology. Its overarching questions are not about facts of the natural world but of meaning, especially of meaning in the human social world. Its contributions do not compete with scientific explanations of how things work. The Bible and its descendent interpretative traditions—rabbinic Judaism, Christianity, and Islam—offer possible meanings for why things work as they (appear to) do. Because they attend to different kinds of questions altogether, biblical and religious texts generally are thus complementary to scientific investigations and philosophical meditations.

Eating is a prime example. Eating is so fundamental to humanity that the Bible's stories of humanity's beginnings include eating.[2] Indeed, eating is so important that nearly all other kinds of ethically fraught relations and activities are absent in these origin stories. Murder, sexual licentiousness, slander—all pale in significance, it seems, compared to eating; those appear only later in the Bible, thus serving as literary evidence of the physical reality that such moral concerns are intelligible and can be attended to only after we first have gone through the physical and moral issues involved in eating.

Even though many readers are familiar with the following biblical stories, I review them closely to highlight just how critical the Bible considers eating. Before beginning, however, I should explain my approach to these stories. I understand the Bible to be a text that spoke volumes to the ancient world into which it initially emerged. That audience of old felt its various stories to be powerful and important enough to keep track of them and teach them generation after generation. In time, these stories were redacted and written down, and those in turn were stitched together into larger collections: Genesis, Exodus, and the like. These larger chunks were then compiled into what we now know as the Bible. This patchwork emergence of the Bible has been a growing theory of biblical scholars for the past two centuries. It explains in part the presence of multiple authorial voices in the material, perspectives that have different names for God, that focus on dramatically different concerns and populations, that are internally consistent yet inconsistent in relation to other authorial voices, that offer different chronologies. In brief, the Bible as it has been bequeathed to us is a concatenation of sources from different times and climates, cultures and tribes. It is for this reason that I tease apart these various stories.[3]

As is well known, the Bible opens with several stories about how the world and humankind in particular came into being. These stories situate eating as a—if not the—primal moral concern confronting humankind. Eating is built into the very structure of human existence; it is an ontological concern. Many biblical scholars point to other important features in these stories about the world's origins and humankind's supposedly superior situation within it. While those details have long shaped such human attitudes and practices as human treatment of animals and stewardship of the environment, not to mention gender relations, eating receives much less attention. I aim here to reclaim eating's central role in creation.

Several versions of creation exist in the Bible, and each contends with eating in a prominent way. The first, Genesis 1:1–2:4a (which I will call Creation One), is perhaps the most famous: in a very orderly fashion God speaks the cosmos into being, and the last creatures spoken into existence are humans. The second version, Genesis 2:4b–3:24 (Creation Two), is dramatically different. Instead of only speaking, here God actively makes the stuff of the world, including the Garden of Eden, and forges humankind early on in the process. Though infrequently considered a creation story, the Noah chronicles of Genesis 6:9–9:17 (Creation Three) nevertheless articulate a revitalized world in which humankind features prominently. Careful reading of these three creation stories reveals eating as a common thread, but their treatment of this critical topic differs.[4] Even as these distinctions need to be appreciated, eating is shown consistently as humanity's first and foremost existential and moral concern.

## CREATION ONE

God, whose name in Creation One is *Elohim*, speaks quite often, and this divine speech has extraordinary power. Above the waters of the deep, "Let there be light," God says, and lo, there is Light. There is evening and there is morning, a first day. Next God speaks into existence vast expanses amid the abundant water, and Sky is created. Then by divine utterance dry land juts above waves, creating Earth and Seas. Then vegetation upon that land is spoken into existence. Then stars, sun, and moon are told to take their places in the expanse of the sky. On the fifth day God speaks forth creatures in the waters, flying birds, sea monsters, and other creepy crawly things. God blesses these creatures, saying, "Be fertile and increase, fill the waters in the seas, and let the birds increase on the earth."[5] On the sixth day God invokes land creatures into the scene. God organizes these animals according to their species based on their habitats: cattle, creeping things, beasts of the earth.

The story crescendos to the moment God speaks humankind into existence with perhaps some of the most famous words in the whole Bible: "And *Elohim* said, 'Let us make humankind in our image, after our likeness. They shall rule the fish of the sea, the birds of the sky, the cattle, the whole earth, and all the creeping things that creep on earth.' So *Elohim* created humankind, in [God's] image [God] created him; male and female [God] created them."[6] For thousands of years, people have fixated upon and wondered why God speaks in the first-person plural, what the difference between "image" and "likeness" is, what is meant by dominion over animals and nature generally, and the egalitarian nature of the concomitant creation of the sexes. These are fascinating and important questions, but watch what comes next: God blesses these new humans with something strikingly similar to that which was bestowed upon the creatures just the day before.

> *Elohim* blessed them, and *Elohim* said to them, "Be fertile and increase, fill the earth and master it; and rule the fish of the sea, the birds of the sky, and all living things that creep on the earth." *Elohim* said, "See, I give you every seed-bearing plant that is upon all the earth, and every tree that has seed-bearing fruit; they shall be yours for food. And to all the animals on land, to all the birds of the sky, and to everything that creeps upon the earth, in which there is the breath of life, [I give] all the green plants for food."[7]

Food is part of the world from the beginning, though not all of the world is meant to be eaten. On the one side God is the provider of food, and on the other are eaters: animals and humankind. Despite the possible complaints of carnivores and some omnivores, if God prescribes this vegetarian—no, frugivore or vegan diet—it must by definition be good and healthy for one and all.[8]

Though all creatures are restricted to consuming a particular kind of food, God grants them permission to eat without any quantitative restrictions. We denizens may eat as much of this fare as we like, as much as we can stomach.

This limitless consumption has a purpose, of course: humans, like their other animal counterparts, are to eat so they can procreate. Note the two instances of "God said" in the quote above. The first divine saying articulates God's blessing to procreate; the second focuses on God's provision of adequate food. The former is the goal, the latter the means. However aloof God may seem in this creation story, God certainly knows biology's requirements: organic beings need constant energy intake. It would be impossible to fulfill the divine blessing to increase and multiply with only the resources already internal to creatures' organic bodies. All creatures—humans, animals, and even vegetation—need additional resources to grow, increase, mature, procreate. All must take from the world in order to be and to make more.

Without eating, we could not fulfill the blessing. Without eating we would not have the energy to conceive another body, much less nourish it adequately. At another level, without eating we would not be able to conceive or perceive another thought, such as fulfilling this very blessing, as we would be consumed with our own hunger. Without taking in additional energy, we would have nothing to give mentally or bodily. Without taking into ourselves what is beyond ourselves, we could neither fulfill nor comprehend our blessing. The blessing is possible, is intelligible, only *after* eating.

Eating here is thus predominantly utilitarian. It enables us to reach not just random goals but the idealized one God signals as appropriate, as primal and fundamental for us: begetting yet another generation. We are to eat to procreate. According to this story, eating is structured and organized. Each creature eats the food appropriate for it: fruit and vegetables for humans, greens for everything else.

Today some might say that we have fulfilled God's blessing: humans run rampant on all continents and are multiplying so quickly that we are stripping the carrying capacity of many of our habitats, perhaps even of the whole world. We have filled the earth, they say, so we should slow down on pursuing the blessing of bearing more children. Others strongly disagree, insisting that God's blessing indicates no limit. Deliberately curtailing our procreative activities would be contrary to God's will. Our progeny should be boundless. This latter mind-set has dominated biblically influenced civilizations for the past several millennia: we may eat ad nauseam to reproduce ad infinitum—despite the fact that the earth already groans in part because of our zest to multiply.

Copious amounts of food and boundless progeny are not the ultimate end of Creation One, however. Rather, this story concludes with God ceasing the work of creation. God rests and blesses this final day of rest.[9] The Sabbath is a holy day because in it creation and its various proliferating creatures can just *be*. This temporal pause completes, reflects, and reinforces the rhythm of the whole story: what is spoken into being in each day just *is*. The story ends with everything stopping; there is no movement, there is no *more*. Creation One neatly culminates in blessed stasis. *Amen*.

## CREATION TWO

The second creation story (Genesis 2:4b–3:24) is messier than the first. Here God, whose name is *Adonai Elohim,* is comparatively quiet yet far more actively creative. The first thing this God does is forge a human by combining dust of the land with Godly breath. This concoction of organic material combined with divine *ruaḥ* (Hebrew for *pneuma*, breath) is rightfully called "a living being."[10]

God plants a garden in Eden in the East and places into it this newly fashioned human. No generic monocrop, this garden abounds with various species: "And from the ground *Adonai Elohim* caused to grow every tree pleasing to the sight, and good for food, with the tree of life in the middle of the garden, and the tree of the knowledge of good and bad."[11] From the start, at least three different plant species exist: those that are aesthetically pleasing, those that are nutritious, and those that are peculiar—the tree of life or immortality and the tree of (the knowl-edge of) morality. Why? Why so many kinds of plants? Why these kinds in particular?

About this diversity the text says nothing just yet. Instead, God now speaks for the first time directly to the human newly situated in this glo-riously divine arboreal idyll. God's first words to this new human are not subtle. For the first time ever, God explicitly commands: "Of every tree of the garden you may eat, but as for the tree of the knowledge of good and bad, you must not eat of it; for as soon as you eat of it you shall die."[12] Similar to the first creation story, this divinely stipulated diet is vegan. But whereas divine speech in Creation One *does* things—creates stuff of the cosmos, bestows blessings upon certain creatures, and grants food—here in Creation Two, God's utterance enables by *commanding* eating as such. Yet, God's words impose restrictions on that consumption and in-troduce the very concept of consequences for noncompliance. Curiously, the prohibition here concerns only one of the two peculiar trees—the tree of moral wisdom—suggesting that it matters more, theologically speak-ing, than all others. (The other peculiar tree—the tree of immortality—is only later identified as out of bounds.) Whereas the first story promotes unrestrained eating, or *ad libitum*, this one clearly constrains. Something about consumption is dangerous here, and God cautions humankind to pay attention to this fact. Eating cavalierly is existentially, even theologi-cally hazardous.

Let's be clear: while eating is God's first and foremost concern here and not procreation, eating is not God's only concern about and for humankind.

Having forewarned the primordial man, Adam, to eat carefully, God nonetheless worries about the man's loneliness. So God endeavors to cre-ate a suitable partner for him. All the animals that God trots before the man fail to pique his interest much less satisfy him. Only when God forges a novel creature from the man's own flesh, a woman, does Adam declare his existential loneliness ended. To her he cleaves.

Naked, unashamed, partnered, surrounded by a divine cornucopia—what could go wrong? A great deal, as we know.

Now another creature appears in the story: the *nahash*, commonly yet mistakenly understood to be a serpent.[13] This *nahash* speaks with the

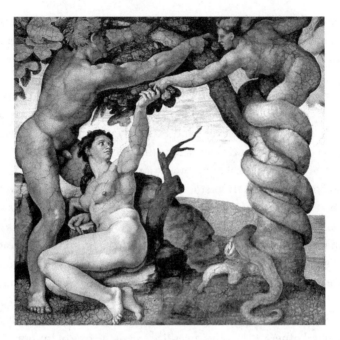

**FIGURE 6.1**

Buonarotti Michaelangelo, *The Fall and Expulsion from the Garden of Eden*, detail at the Sistine Chapel, 1509–1510.

woman in a now famous conversation.[14] We would do well to revisit that conversation, since eating has a central role therein:

> The *naḥash* said to the woman: "Did *Elohim* really say, 'you shall not eat of any tree of the garden?'" The woman said to the *naḥash*, "Of the trees of the garden we may eat. But of the fruit of the tree in the middle of the garden, *Elohim* said you may not eat from it nor touch it lest you die." The *naḥash* said to the woman, "You are not going to die, for *Elohim* knows that as soon as you eat from it and your eyes are opened, you will be like gods [or, like *Elohim*] knowing good and bad." The woman saw that the tree was good for eating, and it was a delight to the eyes, and the tree was a pleasing source of wisdom—she took of its fruit and ate. She also gave to her husband who was with her, and he ate. The eyes of both of them were opened and they knew they were naked, and they sewed together fig leaves and made for themselves loincloths.[15]

The *naḥash* both agrees and disagrees with God. On the one hand, it concurs that a fundamental connection between eating and moral knowledge exists. Yet contrary to God's pronouncement, consuming this peculiar tree's fruit does not induce immediate death. Behold: since the woman and the man survive the moment of consuming from that supposedly deadly tree, the *naḥash* apparently tells the truth, and God had not. Does this mean God lied? Perhaps, or maybe God merely (and certainly purposely) failed to reveal the whole truth in the first instance.

Divine lies aside, something even more powerful hides within this story. The woman seemingly misunderstands God's eating prohibition. She incorrectly says that the fruit of the tree in the middle of the garden is forbidden to consume. When the text describes the garden's layout, however, the centermost tree is the tree of immortality, not the tree God forbade to the humans. God explicitly prohibited them from eating the fruit of the tree of moral knowledge. And since this peculiar tree is not in the orchard's center, it could be anywhere. No human could know precisely where this arboreal source of moral knowledge is situated. She certainly could not know this since the prohibition of eating from that tree was told to Adam before her own creation. She must have come to learn about the prohibition secondhand, from Adam. Either he conveyed the content of God's message accurately, including this vague prohibition of an unidentified and unidentifiable tree, or he himself was unsure what God meant and mixed it all up when teaching her God's rules about eating. Regardless, hers is not an act of disobedience as much as one of misunderstanding. Whose responsibility this misunderstanding is remains an open question.

However mistaken she may be about the tree of immortality, she is quite certain about the tree of morality. Whereas all other trees are *either* nutritious *or* appetizing, in her eyes the tree of morality is simultaneously nutritious *and* appetizing *and* a source of desirable wisdom—so wholesomely enticing, anyone not wanting to eat of it would be a fool. Being no fool, she takes from it and eats. Apparently it is such an abundant source she gives some to her nearby yet strangely silent husband. (Why doesn't he speak up and correct her misunderstanding? What is he afraid of? The dynamics of gender, food, knowledge, power, and relationships are obviously ancient.)

The quality of this arboreal source of divine moral wisdom is questionable, however. Immediately after eating its fruit and as soon as God asks where they are, the man evades the question, and when God asks if they ate from the forbidden tree, the man blames the woman and the woman blames the *nahash*.[16] If they are truly endowed with divine *moral* wisdom, why do they deny responsibility so quickly, as if they are immature? Is this really what morally divine beings do? On the contrary, avoiding accountability wherever and however possible is what the shrewd do. Having eaten of the tree of the knowledge of morality, these humans become even more cunning and crafty than they had been. They hide themselves both verbally and physically, under diversions and loincloths, behind bushes and above blame.

But God is no lazy fool either and finally catches up with the cowering humans. Divinely discovered, everyone is in trouble now: the *nahash*, the woman, the man. Rules have been broken. Improper eating has happened. Consumption of (dubious) moral knowledge has occurred. Awareness of shrewdness and nakedness has spread. Untruths have been spoken. Clothes have been made. Though death was initially divined, it is oddly absent.

Oy.

As if struggling to regain control of a bad and worsening situation, God doles out consequences. The *nahash* now becomes accursed, more than even the cattle and wild beasts: it must crawl upon its belly and eat dirt and suffer the animosity that will forever exist between it and womankind. (This new morphology and diet now make it reasonable to view the *nahash* as a serpent, correlative with other naturally occurring serpents.) God curses the woman with painful childbirth and makes her subservient to her husband. The man, God says, must now labor mightily to extract nourishment from the fields until he eventually and inevitably returns to the ground: "For from it you were taken, for dust you are and to dust you shall return."[17]

Insofar as these divine consequences are to have theological significance, they must radically change the ontological character of these creatures. Accustomed to securing nourishment easily from God's garden, the man must have been wholly ignorant of his ultimate demise and dissolution into the very dust from which he must now extract his nutrition. This does not mean that he was not going to die, just that he did not know that he was. Earlier, the woman could have given birth without pain and had no need to kowtow to her husband; indeed, didn't he follow her lead? Earlier the *nahash* had such amicable relations with the woman it could eat and converse with her even about divine topics, and their conversation was not so unusual that the man felt he had to intervene.

Are these consequences truly punishments? They could be, or they may be theological "just so stories" or etiologies. They are religious explanations of how things came to be, not how they must be.

Consider the final verses to this story.[18] After meting out these consequences God muses that lest these humans again eat food outside the realm of the permissible and specifically from the tree of immortality and thereby become like gods, as the *nahash* surmised, it would be best for them to be escorted out of the Garden of Eden altogether. God thus deposits them beyond the garden's borders, leaving them to forge a life for themselves in the wilds and laboriously extract food from the dusty land even as they form a new relationship together. Unlike Creation One's fixation on procreation and culmination in rest, Creation Two concludes with relation and work.

Still, one overarching theme or concern weaves throughout this creation story. It is not infidelity, murder, abuse of power, fraud, slander, sexuality, narcissism, procreation, or even idolatry. The issue that exercises God and consequently humankind is what and how to eat. Eating is not *a* but *the* fundamental—theological and ontological—issue around which humankind's creation orbits.

## CREATION THREE

The third creation story is even more troubling.[19] It begins not with the world's creation but with its unmaking and only thereafter its reemergence: destruction begets creation. Here God (*Elohim*) regrets creating the miscreant humans and plots to blot them out with all the other creepy, beastly, and flying denizens.[20] God singles out one human, Noah, because of his relative righteousness and informs him of the divine destructive plan. God instructs him to build a mighty ark into which he must bring two of each species, along with his wife, sons, and daughters-in-law.

But that is not all Noah is to bring with him. God continues, "For your part, take of everything that is eaten and store it away, to serve as food for you and for them."[21] Mere bodily escape from the promised deluge is insufficient; provisions also must be secured before God would, or perhaps could, destroy the world. Noah, himself an imperfect human, is now responsible for providing nutrition for all. He must somehow squirrel away more than what is necessary for a picnic lunch. Depending on the version of the story one reads, he must gather enough food to feed everyone and everything for 40 or 150 days of rain, as well as for another 54 to 220 days once the rains stop and the waters begin to subside. In brief, he needs to collect enough food for all creatures upon and within the ark for anywhere between a quarter and a whole year. Gathering so much food is one thing, and cramming it into the ark is another, but maintaining that vast quantity for so long without the benefit of refrigeration or other modern preservation techniques is miraculous indeed.

So even before the rain falls, the world is curiously upside down and inside out. Noah salvages and nourishes creation's beings while God seems hell-bent on wrecking completely everything that humans have spoiled. Here a human saves and feeds while God damns and destroys. Yet just as God planned, the rains come and right the regretted wrongs; the world can begin afresh, and so can eating.

When the flood is over, God instructs Noah to disembark so that the teeming animals and birds and creepers can "be fertile and increase on earth."[22] With strong echoes of Creation One, God blesses Noah and his sons at length:

> Be fertile and increase, and fill the earth. The fear and dread of you shall be upon all the beasts of the earth and upon all the birds of the sky— everything with which the earth is astir—and upon all the fish of the sea; they are given into your hand. Every creature that lives shall be yours to eat; as with the green grasses, I give you all these. You must not however, eat flesh with its life-blood in it. But for your own life-blood I will require a reckoning: I will require it of every beast; of man, too, will I require a reckoning for human life, of every man for that of his fellow man. Who-

ever sheds the blood of man, by man shall his blood be shed; for in [God's] image did God make man. Be fertile, then, and increase; abound on the earth and increase on it.[23]

Once again the primal goal is to multiply. Once again God acknowledges that humans must eat to produce progeny.

Yet something is radically different now. The first creation story grants humans a vegan diet to fulfill the divine vision. To be sure, other creatures surrounded the two primordial humans, but those animals were neither conceived nor perceived as edible. This was true as well in the bucolic garden of the second creation story. This time, however, God gives the few surviving humans permission to consume not just plants but living creatures as well. Flesh is now on the menu.

In addition to this qualitative difference, a quantitative distinction between these regimens exists. Whereas in the first two creation stories the humans were given unfettered access to their diet and could eat as much as they desired, such consumptive freedom is not granted here. God now places explicit and implicit restraints on this new regimen.

When the text says "Every living creature that lives shall be yours to eat," it clearly permits humans to eat any and all animals: the iguana and the alpaca, the dingo and the imperial penguin, the blue whale and the hummingbird. Yet humans may not eat the whole animal. Viscera, muscle, bone, skin, and brain may be consumed, but not blood, based not on biology, though such a reason can easily be concocted since blood is a critical "life force" enabling creaturely animation,[24] but because God said so. Per God's words, shedding blood is such a significant act that no less than God will pursue the one who spills it to extract a "reckoning," whatever that means. I should underscore this point: this text does *not* say spilling blood—animal or human—is inherently bad. God cares deeply about it, but however much concern God may have about blood, God deputizes humans to punish lethally those who shed human blood, a phrase commonly understood to mean murder. God would rather not spill additional human blood directly.

Fascinating! Something about flesh and blood in particular apparently cause God profound discomfort. God explicitly and blandly states in the blessing given to Noah that all animals are "yours to eat." Yours, not

God's. If you humans desire to consume animals, you may do so. But eating animals is a messy business, so you must be careful lest you consume animal blood. Why? Because I, God, said so.

Not unlike God, humans are uncomfortable eating flesh and blood, as is evident in the words we use to name our fleshy food today. A cow becomes *beef*, a pig *pork*, calf *veal*. The former we do not deign to eat, but the latter we eagerly purchase, cook, and consume. Such rhetorical distancing enables a profound unknowing, a willful ignorance by which we assuage our anxieties about consuming animal flesh. Poultry is the one exception: chicken we call *chicken*, duck *duck*, turkey *turkey*. What would happen if we called that sizzling bacon "a sizzling pig" or that hamburger "a cow on a bun"? Why should our words mask our meals?

Now compare God's anxiety about flesh and blood to the next few words: "As with the green grasses, I give you all these." The distinction is stark. On the one hand God does not directly give the animals over to humans to eat but merely says they may be thought of as human food and may be (partially) consumed. On the other hand, what God directly provides and apparently prefers is a vegan diet. Humans may choose to consume animal flesh, though God will not have much to do with it. Because God both distances Godself from punishing lethally those who shed human blood and dissociates from those who voluntarily choose to consume animal flesh, we see that the very idea—and act—of dealing so intimately with creaturely flesh and especially blood troubles God. In a way, spilling blood mortifies God.

*Elohim*, that is. *Adonai*, by contrast, appears less disturbed by animal flesh and blood. When he disembarked from the ark, Noah set up an altar to *Adonai* and sacrificed upon it some clean animals and birds.[25] *Adonai* smelled the *re'ah nihoah*, "pleasing odor," and said inwardly, "Never again will I doom the earth because of man, since the devisings of man's mind are evil from his youth; nor will I ever again destroy every living being, as I have done. So long as the earth endures, seedtime and harvest, cold and heat, summer and winter, day and night, shall not cease."[26] The smell of seared flesh and boiling blood pleases *Adonai* to such an extent that *Adonai* willfully commits to ensuring that Earth's natural cycles will continue indefinitely so that "seedtime and harvest"—essentials for human nourishment—never cease. The smell of a good clean barbecue apparently appeases *Adonai* despite humankind's deviousness. Note that Noah did not partake of any of these animals: they were completely immolated upon the altar. At least for *Adonai*, humans could shed animal blood for proper worship of God but not for human consumption.

The blessing given to Noah by *Elohim* a few verses later similarly articulates in no uncertain terms that humans should pay careful attention to what and how to eat. Blood in particular is viewed as a precious commodity; none shall either spill it or consume it. Because God (*Elohim*, at least) explicitly links murder to the intake of blood, serious consequences logically await both. In brief, if one chooses to eat flesh, eat very carefully.

Drinking also features significantly in Noah's story, but now with a strong echo of Creation Two. *Elohim* declares the rainbow a sign of divine and eternal covenantal commitment not to destroy the earth again. Then comes this episode:

> Noah, the tiller of the soil, was the first to plant a vineyard. He drank of the wine and became drunk, and he uncovered himself within his tent. Ham, the father of Canaan, saw his father's nakedness and told his two brothers outside. But Shem and Japheth took a cloth, placed it against both their backs and, walking backward, they covered their father's nakedness; their faces were turned the other way, so that they did not see their father's nakedness. When Noah woke from his wine and learned what his youngest son had done to him, he said: "Cursed be Canaan; the lowest of slaves shall he be to his brethren." And he said: "Blessed be *Adonai*, the God [*Elohei*] of Shem; let Canaan be their slave. May God [*Elohim*] enlarge Japheth, and let him dwell in the tents of Shem; and let Canaan be a slave to them."[27]

The parallels to Creation Two are plenty: the two names of God (*Adonai* and *Elohim*); Noah, like Adam, is a tiller of the soil; Noah, like God, curses those who should have known better. Perhaps most significantly, the two stories share an overall structure: improper consumption leads to profound and dire consequences.

From one angle, Noah exhibits sophisticated knowledge. Grapes were a sensible crop. The terrain he was on was not a river-irrigated plain on which grains like barley or wheat could readily thrive (these were the main crops in later neighboring civilizations in Mesopotamia and Egypt, and because of this their predominant drink was beer); he was on a mountainous hillside ideal for vines that require little to no additional water. Grapes could supply him with essential nutrients, and their juice could be drunk or made into vinegar. If he was careful—and obviously he was—their juice could be processed into wine. More: because wine, like beer, was a potable and portable liquid, it could be a durable way to quench his and his family's thirst in this new and strange land. Though it would take him a while to do this, of course, since years would need to pass between planting, pruning, plucking, pressing, and vatting, his vineyard would nonetheless supply his family with good drinks for generations. Very smart indeed.

Yet, from a different perspective, though Noah knew how to produce wine, he obviously did not know or understand how to consume it. He became so drunk he passed out in an unsightly manner. His excessive indulgence betrayed his lack of knowledge.

The reason Ham merited Noah's curse was because he saw his father's nakedness. Though the text says nothing about prohibiting seeing a father's nakedness (until much later, halfway through the book of Leviticus), the story presumes that everyone knew the rule, much as in Creation Two it is assumed that Eve knew the rule about the tree of moral knowledge even though she was not there when it was initially promulgated. It was expected that one's physical body would remain unseen, even when asleep or, in this instance, in a drunken stupor. This breech of privacy apparently warranted Noah's outburst toward his three sons (much as God spoke out against the three in the Garden of Eden). His wayward son Ham he cursed with lowly servitude, and to his other sons who did not witness his nether parts he bequeathed prosperity and security.

It could have been otherwise: had Noah not drunk himself into a stupor, his son would not have (unwittingly or not) seen him exposed nor merited punishment. Ham, too, could have received the hopeful future given his brothers. Put conversely again: drinking excessively carries with it dangers for the one who has consumed too much as well as for those who are nearby. The story slams home its moral with a sermonic flair: unrestrained alcoholic consumption damns people and damages families.

Eating and drinking thus play prominent roles both immediately before and after the deluge. Like existential bookends, they envelope the very re-creation of the world. Eating, and now drinking, have become more complicated than in the other creation stories: they are knotted with permissions, restrictions, expectations, and repercussions. Whereas before the flood Noah had to provide all food for all eaters, afterward God ensured there would be food and Noah was free to add flesh to that bounty. If beforehand Noah only had to calculate how much food to bring aboard the ship, afterward he had to be careful about eating certain kinds of food, animal flesh in particular.[28] Before the rains swelled upon the land, quantity mattered in regard to eating; after the waters subsided, quality reigned. Whereas God provided potable rain before and during the flood, afterward Noah took it upon himself to make his own drink within which swirled profound dangers when consumed without conscientious restraint.

In this new world order, eating and drinking require more—not less—attention, vigilance, intention.

## THE GENESIS OF FOOD

Indisputably, eating pervades creation. Each creation story situates eating as so fundamental to human existence that we cannot think of our origins without also considering our nourishment. The stories do this in different ways. Eating in Creation One has a basic biological purpose: it empowers procreation, and all creatures, animals and humans alike, share this consumptive need. In Creation Two, eating distinguishes humankind from all other creatures, such as the *nahash*. It demarcates the genesis of moral and mortal humanity. Creation Three insists that human eating requires forethought, insight, and discipline.

These stories also identify the category of the edible, albeit differently. In Creation One the humanly edible includes only seed-bearing plants; animals are also to eat green plants. All living creatures thus are to subsist on vegetable sustenance. We can surmise from this story that there is a portion of the flora that is off limits to both humans and animals. It could be out of bounds because it is inherently dangerous, but then again, danger is not a concept introduced in this story. Or it could be impermissible just because God never permitted it; it could very well be nutritious food but humankind should never consume it. Regardless, we learn in Creation One that we may eat of the world but not the whole world. Food's ultimate purpose is utilitarian: it enables us to procreate.

Creation Two similarly divides the world into the edible and nonedible. The description here is richer than in the first version. Now the edible world, still populated by only vegetarian beings, includes the nutritious, the desirable, and the off-limits. Linked to these kinds of food are consequences. Some foods enhance, others please, and a few endanger. The themes of tending and tilling and of taking and sharing suggest that food's purpose is relational; when done well, food and eating connect creatures. Improper eating, however, severs or perhaps only severely damages humankind's relation with God: the couple are escorted off the garden's premises with the promise (or curse, depending whom you ask) that only through their own sweat and toil will the soil give forth nutrients necessary for their survival.

Food in Creation Three begins as a purely vegetarian category, but after the flood it comes to include animals. Now recognized as a potentially edible thing, blood is both on and off the menu. It is on for those who would risk dire consequences, and off limits for the rest of us. As in the first story, food's purpose is to empower humankind to produce progeny.

Each creation story thus divides the world that is "not us" into the edible and the nonedible, that which we can and cannot eat, and that which we should and should not eat.


## DIVINE HUNGER

Eating pervades creation. Humans' need to consume the world around them is a common theme that concerns every rendition of the beginning of all things. But food and the need to eat are not just earthly concerns, issues only for mortals to worry about. These are matters of divine concern.

Each story demonstrates God's profound concern about human hunger. Our hunger gnaws at God. We know this because God could have ignored our rumbling bellies. God could have done a great many other things than provide food and offer instructions about good and proper eating. God could have spun off to create other worlds, planted only volcanoes to consume us, laughed at our meager vulnerability. But no. Our hunger haunted God so much that God made sure ample food was available. Such hospitality God provided with alacrity; nothing distracted God in any instance: food and eating are mentioned almost immediately after humankind's emergence on the earthly scene.

Just as hunger is a theological matter, humans also respond to the hunger of others.

Consider that the named humans in these stories also respond to others' hunger. Eve took that fateful fruit and immediately gave some to Adam, and he ate. Noah supplied enough food for his own kin as well as for all other creatures sequestered in the ark. We know all those creatures ate, for when they emerged they came out in droves.

Whether one is providing food for all creation, tasting a particular item, or storing it away for consumption later, it is the other's hunger that one must attend to, as well as one's own. Eating cannot be a solitary and solipsistic endeavor only. Food is food insofar as it is shared. The other and especially the other's hunger commands our attention, and we are to attend to it.

At least three interlocking aspects of eating are thus discernible in these stories. The first creation story speaks of incessant and endless eating, the second of the potential wisdom and relations that eating may engender, and the third of both refraining from consuming the whole animal and excessive alcohol and ensuring that the other has food and enough of it. Strip away eating from creation, and humankind would be neither human nor kind: without eating, how could we be organically, mortally human, and honestly, if we could not feed the other, how could we be morally kind?

Eating is and must be the first physical, theological, and moral issue of human existence. Knowing this fact is vital, for all else follows.

## RATION AND MODERATION

A question left open by these creation stories concerns satisfaction. We learn from these stories that eating is most certainly an existential matter, that food is a divinely circumscribed construct, and that eating anything, fruit or flesh, is an ethically fraught enterprise. What do these stories teach about what it means to eat well? Do they speak about alimentary satisfaction? A preliminary answer hides in moderation: rationing food, eating within bounds.

Return to the Noahide version of creation for a moment. Recall that God instructs Noah to "take everything that is eaten and store it away, to serve as food for you and for [the animals]."[29] To successfully fulfill this mandate Noah would need to know what and how much each animal ate, and then, with the duration of their upcoming voyage in mind, he would need to calculate how much of which food to collect, gather and store it, and be disciplined enough to ration accordingly. If he was sloppy in his calculations or distributed food indiscriminately, he would expose himself and his family to an ugly, hungry, beastly scenario in that bobbing ark. Rationing, then, is critical for existence.

Now venture beyond the creation stories to other biblical material. Consider Moses's instruction to the wandering Israelites as they neared Mt. Sinai, the site where revelation itself would occur. He said they should gather only one *omer* of *manna* per person in a household: "When they measured it by the *omer*, he who had gathered much had no excess, and he who had gathered little had no deficiency: they had gathered as much as they needed to eat."[30] Whereas Noah had to observe what each creature needed to be sustained, Moses (and God through him) exercised authority to dictate what would suffice for each. An *omer* was the basic, and life-giving, ration. Still, both Noah's denizens and Moses's flocks were fed according to a rational rationing system.

Joshua offers a third illustration of a rationing system. He orders the officials of Israel as they are perched above the Jordan River, "Go through the camp and charge the people: get provisions ready, for in three days' time you are to cross the Jordan, in order to enter and possess the land *Adonai* your God is giving you as a possession."[31] The success of this impending theo-politico-military campaign hinged, in part, upon the people ascertaining for themselves what and how much food they should take with them. By not prescribing how much to collect per person, Joshua democratized this task to the population, and its import could not be more significant. Their attention to eating would surely impact the fulfillment of a divine promise, indeed the promise of redeeming the land of Israel for the people and their progeny.

Rationing is thus undoubtedly linked to creation, revelation, and redemption. Discerning the amount of a ration is the result of careful observation of nature (Noah), some external authority (Moses), or a kind of personal assessment (Joshua). Irrespective of its theological, social, or political impulse, rationing is a communal practice that requires each member to eat in moderation. All those animals had to pace themselves, as did the household members around Moses and Joshua's military campaigners. Everyone had to eat in moderation for them to succeed in getting off a full boat alive, arriving at a place where God readily speaks, or liberating a foreign land. Moderation appears to have profound promise. Its theological, social, and political potential suggests that moderation is also an adaptive consumptive strategy. Yet how does one know when one has reached that stage of moderation? What is moderate consumption? Is it an average, a mean, a standard, a median, a range? Or is moderation more individualized, indeed individuating?

# 7

# SATISFACTION

*The pleasure of eating is the only [sense],*
*when moderately enjoyed, not followed by fatigue.*

—Jean Anthelme Brillat-Savarin, *The Physiology of Taste* (1999)

ources other than religion also encourage moderation. For example, philosophical endorsements abound. Their central questions differ from the ones the biblical material pursued, however. Instead of investigating human origins and the ontology of human eating, philosophy explores what eating expresses. Eating moderately conveys one's virtues; it demonstrates one's humanity. Food science is another field that promotes moderate consumption; it questions how eating satisfies and measures how eating en-joys us.

## TEMPERANCE

In antiquity, the Greeks, like the Hebrews of the Bible, advocated eating moderately. Aristotle's treatment of the topic is particularly noteworthy. For him, eating moderately is an expression of one's virtue. Any virtue exists in a continuum between two vices. At one end is a vice of excess, at the other a vice of defect, and smack in the middle is the desired and moderate virtue. In regard to truth-telling, for example, at one extreme is boastfulness and at the other self-deprecation, whereas the ideal virtue of truthfulness (*alētheia*) exists somewhere between those nasty character traits.[1] Virtues thereby illustrate Aristotle's doctrine of the mean.

When Aristotle applies this doctrine of the mean to the physical act of eating he uses the term *temperance* (*sôphrosunê*) because it deals with experiencing pleasure and pain. On the one hand is the excessive vice of profligacy, or the extreme pursuit of pleasure. At the other extreme is the vice of insensibility, of being deficient in relation to pleasure and pain; since this vice hardly exists he considers it inhuman.[2] He narrows the sorts of pleasure temperance involves to the sense of touch, which includes sex, drinking, and eating, though not taste.[3] One reason for this limited list of pleasures is because we share such pleasures with animals. Our wont, Aristotle admits, is to pursue such common pleasures to the extreme—profligacy—and this is bestial. Whereas plants absorb their nutrition directly from the environment, animals and humans cannot. We creatures must rely upon perceptions, and the sense of touch in particular, in order to ascertain and grasp our sustenance. Temperate eating thus relates to and regulates our very animality.

Human eating need not be beastly, however. As in animals, our natural appetite seeks to replenish our bodily needs. Once satisfied, we no longer need to eat nor have the appetite to eat. Profligates, however, derive pleasure from consuming certain foods and thus overreplenish themselves. They do this because they enjoy particular foods, and each person's preferences are idiosyncratic.[4] Even when not hungry, profligates enjoy eating these particular foods. Aristotle hereby points out that eating entails both physical and mental features. On the one hand, eating to satisfy one's appetite meets the body's basic needs and is pleasurable in and of itself. On the other hand, eating to satisfy one's preferences, that one likes this particular food more than that, occurs even when one is not hungry per se. Such consumption is profligate.

Profligacy is wrongful enjoyment. It occurs either by enjoying the wrong thing or by enjoying the right thing more than one should. (Something similar can be said about idolatry: it is the worship of the wrong god or the wrong worship of the right god. Remember the belly worshippers?) Profligates hold a mistaken view of the pleasures of eating, especially of eating certain preferred foods. At the other extreme, insensibility is not wrongful unenjoyment but the lack of enjoyment altogether, and it too is a mistaken view of the pleasure in eating. Insensible people derive little or no pleasure from eating at all and find nothing pleasant or more pleasant than anything else. Anorexics consume too little, but the insensible (if they exist) hardly perceive the enjoyment eating in and of itself naturally brings.

Temperate eaters enjoy eating. Or rather, eating en-joys or causes joy, since it naturally meets a basic bodily need, and those who are temperate experience and welcome such enjoyment. They value it neither too much (like profligates) nor too little (like insensates).

Aristotle identifies several categories of the edible that temperate eaters enjoy: "But such pleasures as conduce to health and fitness he [the temperate individual] will try to obtain in a moderate and right degree; as also other pleasures so far as they are not detrimental to health and fitness, and not ignoble, nor beyond his means. The man who exceeds these limits cares more for such pleasures than they are worth. Not so the temperate man; he only cares for them as right principle enjoins."[5] Some foods contribute to bodily health while others do not compromise bodily health but are merely consistent with it. Some foods would compromise an eater's dignity because they either would demean or are too costly for and would impoverish the individual. Recall that in Creation Two the categories of food include the nutritious, the appetizing, and the peculiar. Aristotle and the Bible seemingly agree that the edible world includes (at least) the healthy, the desirable, and the oddly powerful. While profligates unreasonably enjoy such sensations and foods, and insensates care too little for food at all, temperate people desire and consume what is appropriate. Temperate consumers may eat unhealthy or costly foods from time to time, but when they do, they do not derive enjoyment therefrom because their index for enjoyment is what promotes bodily flourishing.

This critical point shows that temperate eaters desire and consume what is appropriate. Temperate eaters acknowledge their fleshy, animal nature without unreservedly acquiescing to its impulses. They acknowledge their momentary desires for certain foods yet restrain themselves from submitting to those desires wholesale. They strive to ensure their desires remain preferences instead of mutating into needs that they must have in order to be or exist. Conversely, they eat what they need in the amounts they uniquely need.

In this way, each temperate eater eats uniquely. What enables my body to flourish differs from what your body needs. What I can and should eat, that is, what is appropriate for me, is unique; it is not what you should eat, both in kind and quality of food as well as in quantity.

Because temperate eating is peculiar to each individual, any effort to proclaim or dictate the definition of temperate eating will necessarily be inaccurate for all but a few eaters and perhaps outright dangerous for everyone else. Understandably, then, prescriptive diet plans frequently fail: they fail to take me and my body's peculiarity seriously. They do not see me as me but as a statistic in a spectrum of bodies and body types. Their proposals are not for me as such, but for hypothetical eaters. To be sure, diets may offer some insights about healthy eating, but insofar as their authors have never met me or asked me about my own fleshy peculiarities (e.g., metabolism experiences, food preferences), their prescriptions for me necessarily miss the mark. Following their advice would be disadvantageous, perhaps even deadly.

Immanuel Kant observed something similar to Aristotle's temperance among Muslims when making an argument that bodily flourishing is promoted by individualized sleeping patterns, neither too much nor too little as per the body's needs: "It is the same with [sleep] as with the Mohammedan's moderation of eating. The Moslem believes that it has already been determined at the birth of every person how much he should eat. If he is eating much, he will have consumed his portion, and will have to die early. If he eats moderately, he has food to eat for a long time and, consequently, he will live for a long time."[6] Each individual Muslim is to eat mindfully, which means idiosyncratically, lest each risks morbid and even mortal consequences. Bodily flourishing, indicated by longevity, is best achieved and sustained through what Kant calls moderate eating or Aristotle's temperate eating.

Today we call it eating to sate.

## SATIETY AND SATIATION

A central area of investigation in contemporary food science concerns eating. Its main questions are not why we eat, as this has been answered fairly well over the centuries. We eat because we get hungry, and our hunger emerges as we deplete our internal stores of energy. Other reasons have been added to this list: we eat for emotional reasons, social and environmental reasons, hedonistic reasons, and more. But such reasons per se are not what excites or troubles food science. Rather, what exercises food science is the question of how to keep us eating and, conversely, why we cease eating. If we could only know the mechanisms that lead us to stop eating, we could figure ways to keep us eating all the time, which would be a boon for the food industry and the agricultural industry.

It could be said that food science has succeeded in overcoming many mechanisms that regulate our food intake. Many of us eat nonstop, irrespective of whether we are aware of this or not. We eat and drink despite what our bodies need. We are prompted to do so by many pressures. Some are easily recognizable, like the barrage of advertisements of yummy-looking foodstuffs in every media imaginable, the succulent odors wafting across public spaces, and the so-called restaurants conveniently located that serve easily ingestible foodstuffs. I am wary of calling fast-food stores full-fledged restaurants because, historically, a restaurant meant a food that restores or refreshes.[7] What is offered at these chains hardly does either. That said, food science has most surely helped create a food environment in which apparent bounty surrounds us, and through gimmickry and cajoling we buy into it. Often mindlessly, we eat and drink our way through the days, weeks, months, and years.

Eating, however, is not meant to be a continuous experience. Despite the modern food environment in developed countries encouraging us otherwise, our eating should have breaks. We know this precisely because such food environments, and food science in particular, have to work with creative ingenuity to get us to stop regulating our individual consumption habits. Were we left to our own devices, we would, on the whole, eat in intervals and predominantly only as we need. As discussed earlier, we have internal, endogenous mechanisms that help regulate our food intake.

Food science has taken a hard look at these internal regulating mechanisms and has discerned two kinds of naturally occurring impulses that stop our eating. One is a state, the other a process. The first is what keeps us from eating between meals and is called *satiety*. It begins at the last bite of one meal and ends with the first bite of the next meal. Because it occurs after a meal, it is often called postprandial satiety.

The other is a process that begins with the first bite of a meal and ends with the last bite. Think of two curves on a chart: one hunger, the other satisfaction. At the beginning of a meal, hunger is much more intense or

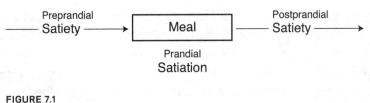

**FIGURE 7.1**

Satiety and satiation.

higher than satisfaction. During the course of a meal, hunger diminishes and satisfaction increases; they have an inverse relation. This process is called *satiation*.

It would not be an exaggeration to say that a central goal of food science is to manipulate both satiety and satiation, interrupting the first and extending the second, so that our eating will become all but continuous from the moment we wake until we fall asleep.

Insofar as satiety is the state of noneating, observing it is fairly easy. Scholarship in satiety centers on the intervals between the conclusion of one meal and the onset of another. Such intermeal intervals indicate that the organism in question is experiencing relative internal stability, or homeostasis. Assessing homeostasis, however, is rather tricky, especially when working with other species with whom communication about their internal states is impossible. But with humans it is possible to get information about how an eater, who is now not eating, is feeling. Human hunger can be communicated. So scientists have asked people to assess and record their subjective experience of hunger after a meal. This subjective variable (called intensity) is coupled with two objective variables: the timed delay of when the next meal is requested (duration) and the amount of food actually taken in during that subsequent meal (the test meal). Putting these variables into mathematical relationships enables scholars to measure satiety ratings, or the motivation to break one's fast and eat again. While earlier studies looked at the next or test meal to calculate satiety ratings, more recent work increasingly attends to the "preload," or the prior meal's energy and weight, since these contribute to the stoppage of eating in the first place.[8]

Such questions also concern satiation because they implicate the various mechanisms that bring a meal to a conclusion. It remains unclear, however, precisely which variables are at play in satiation. For example,

external issues like the weight and energy density of foods impact an eater's intake. So do the environment (physical and social), time pressures
and other stressors, smells (especially those of the foods themselves), and
even how the food is presented (buffet or plated, where on the plate,
course sequence, portion size, etc.). Internal factors of the food itself to
consider are the macronutrient composition of the food, its temperature,
texture, and flavor. Consider, too, factors regarding the eater's act of
eating itself, including the duration of and amount taken in a meal, the
number of bites, the number of chews and swallows, the time taken to
chew, the number and length of pauses, drinks, and more. More factors
include the signals and processes of digestion itself, the distension of the
stomach, nutrient sensors and uptake along the metabolic tract, the regulation of internal energy in the hypothalamus, and short- and long-term
signals of satisfaction associated with the absorption of nutrients.[9] Now
fold in mental states, learned assumptions about what constitutes a meal
and even hunger itself, the anticipation of eating, hedonic or pleasurable
experiences derived from eating in general and eating preferred foods
in particular, and do not forget identity issues like gender, race, class,
education, culture, religion, and more.

All these factors influence satiation. The question of their relative influence remains unanswered, however. Studies show that they influence
satiation in different ways, with different levels of intensity, and at different yet intersecting times. Scholars thus describe a "satiety cascade" of
"successive but overlapping influences" that impact and inhibit eating.[10]

Many of the early studies of satiation were done on animals, especially
rats, dogs, and primates, in laboratory settings, where variables could be
carefully controlled.[11] The physiologist Ivan Pavlov, for one, developed in
nineteenth-century Russia what is now called *sham feeding*. This involves
surgically bypassing the mouth altogether by introducing food and
nutrients lower down in the digestive tract, say, in the esophagus, stomach, duodenum, jejunum, ileum, and even lower down, in the large intestines. Sham feeding, Pavlov found, could keep animals alive and well
nourished, even though they did not derive any flavor or taste from their
sustenance.

Many of us are alive today because of Pavlov's sham feeding studies.
Feeding tubes regularly used in clinical settings build upon his work. We

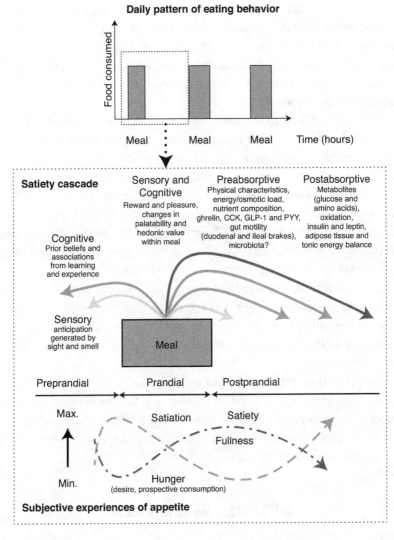

**FIGURE 7.2**

A possible satiety cascade showing waves of interacting factors that influence eating (Sinopoulou et al. 2008).

insert tubes through the nose or skin to deliver water and nutrients at various places throughout the digestive tract. Similarly, we use tubes to remove gastric secretions and partially digested materials so as to mitigate or avoid vomiting, bile buildup, and blockages. By circumventing the mouth and other parts of the digestive tract, we can deliver necessary sustenance and remove waste.

Such interventions in the digestive tract also enable us to observe relations between food intake inhibition—satiation—and gastric nutrient receptors, gastric distention receptors (when the stomach distends as food and drink enter it), gastric emptying, and intestinal and postabsorptive receptors. Bypassing the mouth, tongue, lips, nose, and teeth reveals how our bodies react to foods without being influenced by food temperature, texture, smells, and mouthfeel. Though bypassing the mouth facilitates examination of the internal workings of the gut, one wonders whether such studies get the fullest picture of how eating satisfies.

Even Pavlov himself admitted that full knowledge of eating eluded him. He said it would remain "the subject of ideal physiology, the physiology of the future."[12] Precise and complete knowledge of what happens to food, what food does to the eater, and the features of satiation remain to be determined.

A contributing factor to why our collective knowledge about food and eating is incomplete is that the vast majority of the studies done on these topics share a common assumption, specifically, that the basic eating unit is a meal. Meals dominate even the visual depictions of contemporary theories of satiety and satiation.

## A MEAL IS A MEAL IS A MEAL

Why does the meal dominate our current thinking about eating, and subsequently about satiety and satiation?

The twentieth-century British anthropologist Mary Douglas argues that eating is a kind of code. Codes are languages and can be divided into constituent parts, such as nouns and verbs, and like grammar, relations between the parts can be discerned. Studying eating can thus uncover messages that are encoded therein. In Douglas's view, these messages are essentially social: "The message is about different degrees of hierarchy, inclusion and exclusion, boundaries and transactions across the boundaries. Like sex, the taking of food has a social component, as well as a biological one."[13] These social features of eating can be clarified by linking meals together into an annual chain. Much as words derive their meaning from their immediate and larger contexts, each element in that meal chain derives its meaning from its local and more generic situation.

Douglas defines a meal as solid food accompanied by liquids; "drinks," by contrast, are liquids accompanied by solid foods. In her view, meals are socially more significant than drinks in part because we give them specific names. We have breakfast, brunch, lunch, dinner, supper. The fact that some cultures call a highly ritualized hot drink "tea" can serve as an exception that proves the rule: tea can be had at most any time; lunch cannot.

Another difference between meals and drinks refers to the tools we use. In most cultures meals require mouth-entering utensils, such as forks, chopsticks, spoons. Drinks use mouth-touching utensils: glasses, cups, bowls, straws. Contrasts—temperature, flavor, texture—are more commonly found in meals, whereas drinks are usually all of a kind.

We also impute greater meaning to meals. Compromising one's ability to consume forthcoming drinks is rarely disapproved of, but before a meal it is discouraged. It is more important for the individual body to be primed and ready, that is, hungry, for meals than for drinks. Whom we share meals and drinks with also reflects the relative importance we ascribe to these ingesting events. We are more readily willing to include nonintimates in a round of drinks than we are at meals. Meals we reserve for family, friends, colleagues, known associates, and honored guests. This is in part because drinks facilitate bodily movement. Like the liquids themselves, people having drinks usually stand more than sit. They flow, roam, and bump into each other. Meals, however, are more often taken in a sedentary fashion with movement restricted.

Some anomalous meals challenge Douglas's binary. Picnics, barbecues, and structured cocktail and celebratory parties are a few examples. Still, these exceptions reinforce her contention that meals are infused with great symbolic power.

We can in fact measure a meal as a meal insofar as it incorporates certain features and thus can be contrasted with others in the annual chain. In Douglas's view, our most important or opulent meals are on Christmas, Easter, and birthdays; all other meals may be measured against these. They comprise two basic elements: a main "stressed" course (A) and two side or unstressed dishes (B). These have a similar structure albeit in miniature: a stressed portion (a) and two unstressed ones (b). Her two examples include vegetable soup served with noodles and cheese, and poached eggs on toast with parsley. Each of these would qualify as an A. As in algebra, we can then formulate the meals of the year: Christmas $= A + 2B$, which means one serves a stressed (a+2b) dish and at least two unstressed (a+2b) dishes. By her logic, Sunday brunch $= 2A$; weekday lunch $= A$. Drinks, she says, do not have such structures.

Each meal thus refracts and reinforces the meaning of the whole annual system of meals: "Meals are ordered in scale of importance and grandeur through the week and the year. The smallest, meanest meal metonymically figures the structure of the grandest, and each unit of the grand meal figures again the whole meal—or the meanest meal. . . . The meaning of a meal is found in a system of repeated analogies. Each meal carries something of the meaning of the other meals; each meal is a structured social event which structures others in its own image."[14] For a meal to be a meal it must implicate every other one; it must fit the model. "A meal stays in the category of meal only insofar as it carries this structure which allows the part to recall the whole. Hence the outcry against allowing the sequence of soup and pudding [dessert] to be called a meal."[15]

Would it really be a scandal if soup and dessert were indeed adequate, were considered a meal? Would Douglas's theory of the language of eating crumble, making eating indecipherable? When would a meal not really be a meal?

Two significant criticisms can be levied against studies reliant upon the meal as their basic consumptive unit. The first is something already observed in the 1950s: we tend to eat in units. When given a particular amount of a food or drink, we consider it a unit to be consumed in total. That is, we operate with a "completion compulsion"—an impulse to consume the exact amount served.[16] If given a cracker, we eat the whole cracker; we will drink a full glass of soda when given one. Consuming what is served is called *unit bias* because we are inclined to eat what someone else has already decided to be the proper amount to consume. This tendency to consume easily measurable units of food facilitates the study of eating.

Yet the very definition of the unit has undergone dramatic change in recent decades. Take the simple a+2b lunch of a hamburger, fries, and soda. The U.S. Centers for Disease Control and Prevention found that serving sizes of this kind of lunch have quadrupled since the 1950s.

Not only is the physical quantity of today's meal dramatically larger than it was in previous decades, but its nutritional content has also shifted. This invites the question of whether today's hamburger meal is indeed even a meal. In so many ways it is more than a meal: it is four meals in one.

Obviously, eating by units can be dangerous. Our predisposition to eat units others decide for us and their decisions to expand those very units combine to make a food environment in which overconsumption is easily achieved.

In addition to unit size explosion, another shift in the eating environment that Douglas might consider scandalous is the increasing pervasiveness of snacks. By definition a snack must be a nonmeal, and as such it cannot fit into Douglas's meal chain. Untethered to that system, snacks are left to float throughout our day, crisscrossing our lips in meaningless, socially empty ways, frequently physiologically unfulfilling. Because the companies making them want us to buy and consume more of them, snacks are invariably designed to be unsatisfying and imperfect. Their relative convenience and cost, coupled with their manufactured hyperpalatable qualities, make some snacks virtually irresistible. Many people today pass their days and weeks by consuming snacks almost nonstop. Could snacks be a modern meal, too?

Because a meal is not a constant unit nor composed of consistent elements, the meal is an increasingly contested concept and practice, much to Douglas's chagrin. A meal for some people may hardly register as a meal for others. Whereas one person may indulge in a small snack and call it a meal, another might reserve the name *meal* only for an all-you-can-eat buffet.

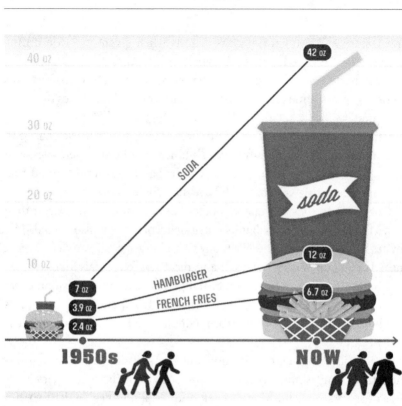

**FIGURE 7.3**

CDC. "The New (Ab)Normal." https://www.cdc.gov/nccdphp/dch/multimedia/info
graphics/newabnormal.htm.

Such variance makes measuring how meals satisfy similarly challenged.
State-of-the-art studies of satiety and satiation increasingly grapple with
these confounding factors for mealtime consumption:

- Social facilitation of eating
- Variations in foods offered
- Palatability
- Sensory-specific satiety and satiation
- Cost and effort necessary to obtain food
- Eating in the absence of hunger
- Environmental ambiance

These and other factors and more influence the amount humans consume at a "meal."[17] Insofar as the very concept of the meal is ambiguous, culturally defined, and ever shifting, relying on it as the basic unit of analysis for satisfaction may be ill-advised. The meal, whatever it means, is an external concept and cue. External, that is, to eaters.

Given that satisfaction is what each eater experiences on the inside, perhaps internal cues would be better benchmarks to measure alimentary satisfaction. Instead of restaurants, companies, nutritionists, or governments deciding what is appropriate or will satisfy, individual eaters should be arbiters of what is appropriate and enjoyable. Temperance, we should recall, is unique to each eater; no outsider can predetermine what would be too much or too little to satisfy each and every eater. Eaters, not feeders, should be the ones to determine what satisfies.

# 8

# JUST RIGHT

*One should hold back before becoming replete.*

—Abu Ḥāmid Al-Ghazālī, *On the Manners Relating to Eating /*
*Kitāb ādāb al-akl* (2000)

The turn to the eater as the measure and measurer of satisfaction can be buttressed by religious teachings about satiation, which invariably insist that each person serves as the ultimate arbiter of what is enough for himself or herself. Enough cannot be prescribed by measuring against some arbitrary concept like a "meal" (e.g., A+2B) or a particular quantity of certain macronutrients. Such ways of thinking and speaking about enough refer to and defer to external cues. They orient eaters to attend more to what is outside of themselves, to the food itself, its qualities, features, and presentation, among other facets, rather than to the eater's own sensations.

Another way to discern satisfaction involves a more internal orientation. The very notion of enough or alimentary satisfaction is perhaps best defined and assessed by each eater from within. For *what* I find satisfying will be unique to me, just as what satisfies you is unique to you. Similarly, *how much* sates me will differ from how much sates you. The only way to figure out what and how much sates is to ask each eater. Overlaps will occur, and this is where our commensal or shared experiences can be rewarding.

No less than a children's story suggests this kind of internal orientation while eating. "Goldilocks and the Three Bears," a ditty of a story originally composed in Britain around 1830, describes a girl (originally an old woman) entering a strange house in the woods. On the kitchen table she finds three bowls of different sizes. Depending on the version of the story, these bowls are filled with such dishes as porridge, milk, or rabbit soup. Hungry, she tastes from each bowl. The largest she finds too hot,

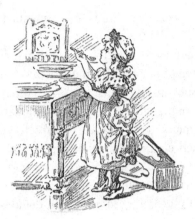

**FIGURE 8.1**

Goldilocks champions a "just right" internal alimentary satisfaction orientation.

which could mean it did not satisfy her because of either its temperature or its spiciness. The middle-size bowl proves to be too cold and tasteless for her palate. The final, smallest bowl, of course, is "just right": it satisfies her completely.[1]

Had Goldilocks a poor understanding of Aristotle's golden mean and reacted to external cues, she would have consumed the middle-size bowl since it was between the extremes. Or if she consumed based on other popular external cues, like cost and convenience, she should have eaten the most of this otherwise free meal: she should have downed the largest bowl. But Goldilocks did neither. She ate what pleased her palate and only as much as satisfied her belly. Her "just right" refers to no external world but to internal cues. Satisfaction emerges from within.

## SATISFACTION

Eating to satisfy oneself can be achieved in several ways: through *quantity*, by eating so much or so little of a food; eating certain *preferred foods*, such as those one likes the taste of or those that are prescribed by a particular dietary regime; or eating *frequently*, by snacking.

Of course, food is necessary to satisfy us gastronomically, but food is only a part of this process. Alimentary satisfaction also has a mental component. This fact was raised early on by Moses in the Bible. He taught the ancient Israelites to distinguish between two kinds of alimentary satisfaction—one dangerous, the other laudatory.

The dangerous kind of satisfaction comes from eating one's fill, enjoying one's bounty, and thinking, "My own power and the might of my own hand have won this wealth for me."[2] Such hubris disregards God's intervention that liberated Israel from their oppression in Egypt. It also downplays that it is God who empowers humans to gather their bounty in the first place. By forgetting God, this self-congratulatory eating attitude leads to the grave, for it embodies the depravity and disobedience God abhors and will eradicate.[3] According to Rabbi Bahya ben Asher ibn Halawa, this kind of irreverent eating is to be eschewed because it deludes eaters into thinking bodily pleasures are an ultimate goal, and thus it verges on idolatry.[4]

The other, more promising kind of satisfaction is more theological in orientation. Moses instructs the Israelites to recall all the amazing things God has done for them, including taking them out of Egypt and guiding them through the desert. What Israel endured was purposeful: "[God] subjected you to the hardship of hunger and then gave you manna to eat, which neither you nor your fathers had ever known, in order to teach you that man does not live on bread alone, but that man may live on anything that *Adonai* decrees."[5] Remember this, Moses says, for "when you have eaten your fill [*ve-achalta ve-sava'ta*], give thanks to *Adonai* your God for the good land which [God] has given you."[6]

Such grateful consumption is simultaneously inwardly and outwardly oriented. Externally, it considers God's role in the fact that one has food to eat at all. Internally, it stresses that each is a singular eater. The Hebrew—*ve-achalta ve-sava'tah*—literally means "you (singular) shall eat, and you (singular) shall be satisfied." The dangerous kind of eating similarly understands people to be unique eaters sating themselves.[7] The difference here is the eater's orientation. This more wholesome mode of eating is not merely for homeostasis and self-aggrandizement; it involves satisfying oneself gastronomically and simultaneously acknowledging that one's very sustenance comes not from the self. Good alimentary satisfaction, then, is what situates one's own body in a larger, interactive context. Rabbi Bahya applauds this kind of eating because it engenders bodily health and intellectual clarity.[8]

One should not eat to be full since self-satisfaction is hardly different from idolatry. Rather, because humans receive free (*gratis*, in Latin) gifts from God like food itself, one should eat to be full of gratitude. Hence, Moses's instructions to give thanks to God.[9]

Yet a critical question remains unanswered in these teachings. *Sove'ah*, or satisfaction, is a powerful concept that can be understood in several ways. What might "eating until one is satisfied" actually mean in practice? As will be shown, eating what is "just right" is satisfying.

## JUST RIGHT

The prophet Elijah never died, according to the Bible. Instead, he ascended to heaven in a fiery chariot.[10] The rabbis fancifully build on this detail by having Elijah appear every now and then in the literature to offer a lesson, observe people's behavior, supervise rituals, and have a chat with this or that person. Amid a larger rabbinic conversation about food remedies for various ailments, Elijah meets with Rabbi Nathan, a second-century sage, to offer this directive: "Eat a third, drink a third, and retain a third."[11]

What does Elijah mean by this? It could mean to eat and drink only a third of what is served and take away the remaining third, or perhaps it means to throw that last third out. Such interpretations are quite plausible if one takes an external perspective.

A more internal orientation offers a completely different meaning. Rabbi Shlomo ben Yitzchaki (also known as Rashi), an eleventh-century French biblical exegete, believes Elijah's comment refers to one's stomach, not one's plate. For Rashi, Elijah means that one should fill one's stomach only a third with food and a third with drink and leave a third of it empty.[12] Eating well is not to be determined by what one sees on one's plate, by external cues, but rather by assessing one's internal cues.

Elijah's lesson does not end here, though. To his two-thirds teaching he adds this rationale: "For when you become angry you will be filled to your capacity."[13] Why should he speak of anger here? To our ear this makes little sense. But to Rabbi Nathan, and all other rabbis of that era, it made perfect sense because they took the prevailing Hippocratic and

Galenic theories of human physiology seriously: they held a humoralist conceptualization. According to this theory, each person's health and temperament depend upon the dynamic balance of four humors: black bile, yellow bile, phlegm, and blood. Any imbalance of these basic building blocks will manifest fleshy ailments and personality disorders. Humoralism's significance cannot be denied: it spread throughout ancient civilizations and dominated world medicine and philosophy up until the nineteenth century or so.

According to humoralism, emotions too are physical. They are a sloshing of these internal fundamental substances, so recalibrating them requires bodily processes. In brief, just like the food one ingests, emotions need to be metabolized. Thus Elijah's instruction to leave a third of one's stomach empty of food is to allow space for emotions like anger to be digested so that equipoise, or physical and emotional homeostasis, can once again be achieved.

Rashi concurs with Elijah and adds this graphic detail. "Anger fills your belly to its utmost capacity. So if you fill your innards with food and drink, when you become angry you will be split asunder."[14] Rashi urges neither sublimating one's anger nor ignoring it altogether. He recognizes that one's emotions are what they are. Emotions must be respected and given ample room to transform. They are part of who one is; they constitute in part one's personality and by extension one's very life. Thus filling one's stomach with biology leaves insufficient room for biography. The consequence of eating until one is full would be lethal.

For Elijah, then, to eat well is to eat more than nothing yet less than one can. This idea was widely embraced throughout the ancient and medieval world. Yet his proposal to consume only until one's belly is two-thirds full met with some surprising emendations.

Moses Maimonides, the great Jewish legist, philosopher, theologian, and physician of twelfth-century Egypt, wrote in a letter sometime after 1193 to al-Malik al Afdal nfir al-Din 'Ali, the son of Saladin, the following medical advice: "Physicians all agree that taking a little food of bad quality is less harmful than taking much good and laudable food. This is because when a man takes bad foods and does not overeat, they are digested well, and the organs derive from them all that is beneficial. . . . But in repletion even if it is with well-prepared bread and laudable meat, the digestion will in no wise progress well."[15] Ease of digestion and bodily health justify eating less than the full capacity of one's stomach. Over a decade earlier, in his legal code, the *Mishneh Torah*, Maimonides offered another reason: "A learned sage should not be a glutton, but should eat foods according to the health of his body, and should not eat overly large meals, and should not rush to fill his belly as do those who fill themselves with food until they burst."[16] According to Rabbi Abraham ben Meir Ibn Ezra, a twelfth-century Spanish philosopher and exegete, wicked people eat hurriedly, perpetually, and gluttonously and are never satisfied.[17] Perhaps Maimonides and Ibn Ezra grounded their positions on the proverb "The righteous eats to satisfy himself, but the belly of the wicked is empty."[18] Regardless, Maimonides holds that sage eating is idiosyncratic (the foods are appropriate for the individual's body), modest (less than complete repletion), and spaced (with meals reasonably paced and separated in time).[19]

Though Maimonides agrees with Elijah that eating well is by definition eating more than nothing and less than one's full gastric capacity, he disagrees with what that ideal amount should be. In his view, "one should not eat until one's stomach is [very] full, but one should [only] eat until one's stomach is three-quarter's full."[20] Elijah's proposal is too stringent for Maimonides. Sage eating, or eating well, need not be so stingy. One should definitely eat more than nothing yet not more than three-fourths full. This range would be just right.

While a bit more lenient than Elijah's, Maimonides's approach carries forward the idea that one needs to retain bodily space to metabolize one's emotional life. This is because he too was a humoralist, believing that meaningful human and humane existence is best achieved by eating what is "just right." Doing so would optimally sustain both one's biology and biography.

Unsurprisingly, Jews were not the only ones to think about what constitutes eating well. Muslims, too, eschewed eating at extremes and embraced eating what they thought was just right. For example, a popular hadith, or saying attributed to Mohammad, teaches, "A man does not fill any vessel worse than his stomach. It is sufficient for the son of Adam to eat enough to keep him alive. But if he must do that, then one-third for his food, one-third for his drink and one-third for his air."[21] The great eleventh-century Muslim philosopher, theologian, and legist Abū Ḥāmid Muḥammad ibn Muḥammad al-Ghazālī acknowledged the popularity of this teaching:

> One of the People of the Book [which could mean either a Christian or a Jew], who was a philosopher and also a physician [this could not be Maimonides, as he was born twenty-five years after Al-Ghazālī died], once heard the statement of the Prophet (Peace Be upon Him), "One third for food, one third for drink, and one third for breath." Astonished, he declared, "I have never heard wiser words than these regarding frugality in eating. These are wise words indeed!" The Prophet (PBUH) once said, "Satiety [meaning surfeit consumption here] is the beginning of sickness and fever the beginning of physic [requiring the care of physicians, such as with leeches, purging, etc.]." It is my opinion that the surprise of the aforementioned physician was at this latter Tradition [that is, teaching], not the former.[22]

Though it may not ultimately matter whether this non-Muslim philosopher-physician was astonished at Mohammad's teaching that excessive consumption causes sickness or his teaching that one should eat less than one bodily can, the two-thirds position had traction among at least Muslims and Jews who harkened to Maimonides.

We should note the reasons supporting these two teachings. The two-thirds ratio is based upon the authority of the Prophet: one should eat this much because he said so. The reason behind not eating too much is physical: eating too much causes sickness, requiring medical attention.

Elsewhere Al-Ghazālī added another set of reasons behind eating just right. He insisted that essential to prophethood and to gain entry into the Kingdom of Heaven one must eat up to one-half of one's stomach's capacity: "Said Abu Sa'id al-Khudri, 'The Emissary of God (PBUH) once said, "Wear your clothes, and eat and drink up to the middle of your stomachs, for to do this is part of Prophethood."' . . . Al-Hasan relates on the authority of Abu Hurayra that the Prophet (PBUH) said, 'Wear garments of wool, and roll up your sleeves, and eat with only half of your bellies; for thereby shall you enter into the Kingdom of Heaven.'"[23] Holy eating, or at least eating for these holy goals, cannot be done by filling

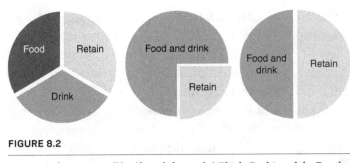

**FIGURE 8.2**

Proposals for eating well by (from left to right) Elijah, Rashi, and the Prophet
Mohammad; Maimonides; Al-Ghazali and the Prophet Mohammad.

one's stomach to its utmost. Nor should it be mostly full. It should not be
empty, either, or have too little in it. Rather, eating to fill half of one's
stomach is most religiously meritorious.

For Elijah and Rashi, eating to fill no more than two-thirds of one's
stomach enables one to metabolize and thus enjoy one's emotional life.
Maimonides insists the compelling reasons for eating up to three-fourths
of one's stomach revolve around physiology and notions of righteousness.
On Al-Ghazālī's account of Mohammad's teachings, the primary motivations include the Prophet's authority, physiology, and theological
rewards. Regardless of their underlying rationales, they all agree that the
proper way to sate oneself is to eat more than too little and less than one's
physical capacity.

Early Christianity similarly embraced the call to eat just right, that is,
to eat less than one can and more than nothing. In John the Baptist's account, Jesus fed five thousand people with just five loaves of bread and
two fish: "Then Jesus took the loaves, and when he had given thanks, he
distributed them to those who were seated; so also the fish, as much
as they wanted. When they were satisfied, he told his disciples, 'Gather
up the fragments left over, so that nothing may be lost.' So they gathered
them up, and from the fragments of the five barley loaves, left by those
who had eaten, they filled twelve baskets."[24] Jesus's ability to feed so many
people is incredible, especially when juxtaposed to a similar incident with
Elijah's prophetic successor, Elisha.[25] Given that Elisha was famous for
providing vital sustenance to the impoverished, for healing the apparently dead, and for changing deadly food into a healthy repast, among

many other miraculous feats, it is not surprising he suggested it was possible to feed one hundred people with just twenty loaves of bread. When his servant wondered how this could be done, Elisha responded, "Give it to the people to eat. Do it because *Adonai* said, "They will eat and have some left over." This is precisely what happened.[26]

Though Elisha and Jesus enact amazing miracles, the people who sit at their feet warrant attention here. The people surrounding them ate until they were satisfied, not until they were stuffed. Even as the people around Jesus took "as much as they wanted," they ate less than that. They ate so that some remained and could be collected. Neither Jesus nor Elisha instructed his guests to eat less than they could, nor did either host provide too much in some kind of ostentatious show. Rather, each person restrained himself or herself from eating all that was made available. Incredible. The miracle in both instances was that the people, individually and collectively, refrained from eating all that was put before them. Good believers eat what is just right: more than too little and less than their full capacity.

## GO AHEAD, REFRAIN

According to these sources, there are strong physical, emotional, intellectual, moral, even metaphysical reasons to eat what is just right. Such motivations are designed to work less on the collective or community and more on the individual. Each person is to consider herself or himself an eater; each is bidden to eat something yet less than one physically can. Go ahead and eat, these sages urge, yet refrain before filling oneself. Why one eats in this "just right" zone is, as I see it, up to each individual. No singular or overriding rationale can or should guide such theological and adaptive eating strategies.

Reconsider for a moment the distinction modern science makes between satiety and satiation. Satiety is the state of noneating between meals; satiation is the increasing inclination to stop consuming a particular meal. Might there be religious analogues or acknowledgment of these kinds of alimentary satisfaction?

The rabbis of the Talmud encourage removing one's hand from a pleasing meal.[27] This admittedly vague teaching avoids stipulating precisely how much one should eat. It does not speak of filling oneself to half, two-thirds, or three-fourths of one's capacity. Rather, it seeks to elicit in eaters the ability and practice of refraining. Even at a meal that delivers pleasure one should refrain from glutting oneself. Satisfaction, it seems to say, derives from *both* the delicious food consumed *and* the very act of stopping before one is full. Go ahead, refrain, and be satisfied.

Maimonides apparently concurs. In his view, "the preservation of health lies in abstaining from repletion and forsaking the disinclination to exertion."[28] Both refraining from stuffing oneself and getting up to exercise are required for vitality. Modern science wonders about this latter stipulation, however. The U.S. National Institutes of Health, for example, have found that exercise alone is insufficient to reduce excess weight or to maintain weight once lost during a diet regimen.[29] Other researchers have found that eating a low-energy diet is more conducive than aerobic interval training at improving insulin-related issues.[30] Even if scientific opinion has not yet reached consensus about exercise, regarding the call to abstain from stuffing oneself, modern science repeatedly finds that calorically restricted diets improve both health and survival in other primates, suggesting something similar for humans.[31] Rashi complements these findings by saying that the little one eats becomes blessed in one's belly.[32] Consuming and then refraining within a meal thus accrues physical as well as sacred benefits.

If these writers speak about satiation, about *stopping* a particular consumptive event before glutting our guts, what about satiety? What, if anything, do they teach about refraining from eating *between* consumptive events?

Maimonides insists "it is one of the rules of the regimen of health not to introduce one meal upon another, and not to eat except after true hunger, when the stomach is empty."[33] Already nearly a thousand years ago people were aware that not eating between meals conduces to health, that we should avoid interrupting satiety with snacks and other mini-meals. Yet we should note that Maimonides stops short of saying precisely what constitutes a break. Breaks between meals must be determined from within, by assessing one's own hunger, and cannot be prescribed from without. External authorities may offer guidelines, but the ultimate arbiter of one's hunger, and what satisfies it, rests on the individual eater.

The importance of refraining within a meal and between them was, for Al-Ghazālī, the highest medical wisdom, as seen in this folklore-like narrative:

> It is told that [Hārūn] al-Rashīd once summoned four physicians: an Indian, a Greek, an Iraqi and a Sawādī [from south-central Iraq], and said, "Let each one of you describe that medicine which itself results in no sickness." The Indian spoke up, and said, "In my opinion, the medicine which contains no sickness is black myrobalan [an herb, typically to treat leprosy]." Then the Iraqi said, "For me, it is nasturtium cress [used to treat leprosy, spleen and menstruation]." The Greek said, "I think it is hot water." And the Sawādī (who was the most learned of them), said, "Myrobalan scours the stomach, and that constitutes a sickness. Nasturtium cress renders the stomach oily, and that is a sickness also. Hot water slackens the stomach, and that also constitutes a sickness." And so al-Rashīd asked him, "Then what is your answer?" And he replied, "In my opinion, the medicine which contains no sickness consists in refraining from food until one has an appetite, and in ceasing to eat when one is yet unsated." "You have spoken truly," he declared.[34]

Just a bit farther on, Al-Ghazālī relates that Ibn Sālim "was asked what the due propriety might be, and [he] replied, 'To eat after the onset of hunger, and to stop before the onset of satiety.'"[35]

When hungry, go ahead and eat. Then, once satisfied, refrain.

Long, then, have humans appreciated what is now known as satiety and satiation. For centuries, millennia even, people have been encouraged to refrain from glutting themselves in any one prandial event or cumulative series of events. Taking breaks between meals and ending a meal before one reaches repletion have long been coupled together.

Eating just right and eating well involve eating enough to sustain oneself and not so much as to compromise one's bodily health, moral uprightness, or religious merit. This kind of eating well requires knowing oneself well enough to know when to start and stop eating.

## JUST RIGHT IS LESS THAN BEST

Let's call being contented by eating less than one bodily can *alimentary satisfaction*. One *could* fill one's stomach with food and drink, but one refrains; according to religious teachings, this is both satisfying and meaningful, and according to modern science, it is a path to improved and sustained health. Put differently, good things come about when one's fullest capacity is *not* reached.

Curiously, studies in social psychology offer similar insights, albeit not associated with gastronomic consumption. Consider, for example, a 1995 project that looked at Olympic athletes.[36] According to that study, those who won bronze medals were, at both the end of a competition and on the awards podium, happier than those who secured silver medals. This counterintuitive observation emerges from counterfactual thinking. Silver medalists tend to think about the individual or team they failed to best. Their counterfactual thinking—"what might have been"—is fixated on that shortcoming. Because they did not win gold they feel low. Bronze medalists, by contrast, rarely compare themselves against those immediately in front of them but with the whole host of competitors they bested. For them, had they not achieved what they did, they would not have received any award at all. Because their comparisons are the "nones," or the ones who received no award at all, they tend to appreciate what they have all the more.

In some competitions, second-place winners are actually losers of the last round of competition and third-place winners are winners of the penultimate round of competition. Such structures no doubt influence the overall satisfaction experienced by silver and bronze medalists. But other forms of competition, such as track and swimming, end in a single-file manner. The same study found that overall satisfaction is consistent across these competitive structures. In brief, silver medalists wrestle with the fact that they *just nearly* missed winning the whole darn race, whereas bronze medalists glory in the fact that they *just barely* got to the podium at all. Put in different terms, being substantially below the best generates more psychological satisfaction than being closer to the top.

Perhaps there is an analogue between psychological satisfaction and alimentary satisfaction. Eating until one has reached repletion has repeatedly been found uncomfortable and soporific. Eating to one's utmost enervates, whereas eating less than one ultimately could counterintuitively energizes. Though Nathan's (the company that sponsors the annual hotdog-eating contest) may not want to hear this, eating is not nor should it be some kind of competition. Just as comparisons are unnecessary for eating well, so too are external judges and goading crowds. Eating is one activity in life in which doing one's best should be between nothing and all-out, or, in this case, all-in. Eating enough is an idiosyncratic task ideally based on internal cues, not external ones. True alimentary satisfaction emerges from within.

Religions have long taught us to eat when hungry and to refrain from eating to our full capacity. Modern science corroborates both practices. When one follows these strictures, one eats adaptively, or just right. It is to eat well.

# IV

# I EAT THEREFORE I AM TASTEFUL

*One cannot think well, love well, sleep well,*
*if one has not dined well.*

—Virginia Woolf, *A Room of One's Own* (1929/1989)

*Out of God's mouth come knowledge and discernment.*

—Proverbs 2:6

# 9

# SAVORING

*What gets eaten must first be tasted—and approved.*

—Leon Kass, *The Hungry Soul* (1999)

*I taste therefore I exist locally.*

—Michael Serres, *The Five Senses* (2008)

Eating well is a moral issue, not just a physical or metaphysical one. Recall Derrida's assertion: "The moral question is thus not, nor has it ever been: should one eat or not eat, eat this and not that, the living or the nonliving, man or animal, but since *one must* eat in any case and since it is and tastes good to eat, and since there's no other definition of the good, how for goodness sake should one *eat well*?"[1]

What does eating well mean given the modern food environment of hyperpalatable foodstuff? What might healthy, adaptive eating be? As it is virtually impossible to prescribe a generic diet that would meet each person's metabolic needs, eating well is idiosyncratic, unique to each person. Nevertheless, some general comments can be made about how eating well today may be achieved.

The chapters in this section discuss some ways eating well or just right can be put into practice. My focus here is on three macronutrients that each person needs for bodily survival. These macronutrients—salts, sugars, and fats—have been brilliantly if not deviously manipulated over the millennia and especially in recent decades to make our foodstuffs so incredibly delicious that resisting them is hard. This chapter investigates why and how these particular flavors are so tasty for us, how manipulating them has been quintessential to our very evolution, and some of the ways consuming them without restraint can be lethal. Chapter 10 digs deeper into reasons to constrain ourselves from eating these particular macronutrients. Religions and biology concur that we should sacrifice unbounded consumption of them. Chapter 11 demonstrates how sharing these and other foods is as good for individuals as it is for communities. We will all do better if we appreciate the fact that we never dine alone.

## *HOMO GASTRONOMICUS* OR *HOMO SAPIENS*?

According to Milton, these were Adam's first words to Eve after consuming the fruit of the forbidden tree of knowledge of good and evil:

> *Eve*, now I see thou art exact of taste,
> And elegant, of Sapience no small part,
> Since to each meaning savour *we* apply,
> And Palate call judicious; I the praise
> Yield thee, so well this day thou hast purvey'd.[2]

Adam does not praise Eve's bodily beauty first, though he certainly lusts for her. Rather, he begins by acknowledging that she is a woman *of* taste as much as she is a woman *who* tastes. Her elegance and sagacity are no less impressive than her discerning palate.

Adam can acknowledge this about Eve because he himself has tasted that forbidden fruit. Knowledge, discernment, and wisdom follow not eating but tasting. Even the wily *naḥash* or Tempter in Milton's essay admits this to Eve:

> Look on mee,
> Mee who have touch'd and tasted, yet both live,
> And life more perfet have attaind then Fate
> Meant mee, by ventring higher then my Lot.[3]

This creature, too, attained wisdom and a life far exceeding fate after tasting the fruit of this tree. As the twentieth-century French American philosopher Michael Serres says, "Wisdom comes after taste, cannot arise without it."[4] Why is this?

Though we often think incorrectly that the mouth is the place where taste occurs, tasting is a synesthetic experience involving multiple senses simultaneously. Tasting integrates sight, sound, touch, and especially smell. We see food on our plate, hear it crackle, feel it in our mouth, crunch it with our teeth, caress it with our tongues. Throughout these experiences, we smell it: as it cooks over there on the stove, as it approaches here on our fork, as it jostles around in our masticating mouth. Indeed, without smell, we could not appreciate flavor in its fullness.

We smell food in different ways, however. One way is externally oriented, the other internally. Orthonasal olfaction, or smelling, that is, breathing directly into the nose, helps us discern healthy from dangerous food as well as the scents of loved ones, the volatile compounds in feces, the bouquet of wine, the smoke of fire. Like sight and hearing, orthonasal smelling senses across distance to help us protect ourselves.

Retronasal smelling, by contrast, ascends from within the body. It carries smells from inside the mouth through the nasopharynx to the nasal cavity. Like its external counterpart, this internal smelling similarly helps protect the body, especially from poisons that have little to no scent when outside the body.

Both exogenous and endogenous smelling bring particles and pieces of the object of concern into the nasal cavity, where they are bodily encountered by the olfactory epithelium and nearly instantaneously mentally analyzed. A critical difference between these kinds of smelling is that orthonasal smelling senses odors, while retronasal smelling produces flavor.

For an easy test to prove the importance of smell to flavor, just hold your nose, take a sip or a nibble of most anything (except water), and try

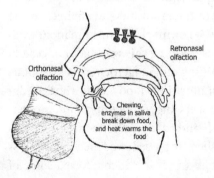

FIGURE 9.1

Orthonasal and retronasal smelling and tasting.

to discern the flavor of what is now in your mouth. With your retronasal smell incapacitated, all you can discern is texture, temperature, and, if you are lucky, some limited taste. With the food or drink still in your mouth, unplug your nose and breathe. This retronasal whiff or puff of air carries particles of the food bolus to your smell receptors that, together with the other sensations from your mouth, combine into what scientists call "the flavor experience."[5]

Neither the mouth nor the nose is the sole site of the flavor experience. Rather, mouth and nose sensations mingle and merge to form the flavor experience in the brain, in no small part because of smelling's significance in our genomic structure. Of the thirty thousand or so genes in our genome, about one thousand, or 3 percent, are olfactory receptors. No other sense—neither hearing, seeing, nor feeling—has as many genes. Relative to other kinds of mammals, like dogs and rodents, however, our ability to sense smell has diminished through evolution. So despite their prevalence in our genome, most (more than 70 percent) of our olfactory receptor genes are actually pseudogenes: they have lost their function.[6] Nevertheless, the physical placement of the olfactory epithelium in our nasal cavity allows it to have direct input to the orbitofrontal cortex area of the brain. This part of the neocortex facilitates the most sophisticated mental faculties, such as language, reasoning, and planning. Smell, evolutionarily speaking, is essential to these aspects of human existence. All other senses go through more complicated pathways to the brain. Smell's genetic dominance and anatomical presence indicate its critical evolutionary importance to sensing flavor, tasting, and eating, indeed to being human.

A plausible reason smell retained its vital contribution to our eating processes and its direct connection to the brain links to changes in the ways we went about feeding ourselves. For much of our humanoid existence, we were like all other creatures roaming this world: our ancestors smelled their way into the future, sniffing out dangerous from safe foods and, if lucky, identifying savory and nutritious foods. Over time we developed other means of detecting dangers and, more important, protecting ourselves. We began to forge tools and engage in collective agency, to name just a few behaviors. As the millennia passed, we relied less and less on our olfactory system to ensure our survival, which allowed some of our smelling genes to fall into desuetude; they became pseudogenes, with no obvious function.

Though we became more microsmatic, or weak smellers, as time went on we became increasingly good at something else, which may be one of the few things that distinguishes us from all other species.

Consider this hypothesis. Our olfactory system clusters close to the brain, much as ancient humans crouched near fires to capture warmth, share stories, arrange tomorrow's hunt, and, most important, cook. Smoky scents intermingled with communication, reasoning, planning, and of course food. Our neurology adjusted to, along with, and for our culinary developments.

Now consider some evidence. The contemporary American primatologist Richard Wrangham demonstrates that the explosive growth of the human neocortex about a million years ago was contemporaneous with human-controlled use of fire for cooking.[7] Why would cooking be related to such significant physiological changes? One possibility is the biological nature of hot food. The heat of cooking breaks down the walls of food cells, lowering the amount of energy needed to digest them. Heat also neutralizes poisons and diseases that the nose and tongue perhaps cannot discern. Heat thus increases the percentage of easily digestible and safe foods for humans. With fewer calories demanded by the gut to do its job, more calories are free to be sent to the increasingly hungry brain. This influx of energy enabled the brain to grow and evolve its newest features, so that today our brain now consumes 20 to 25 percent of our body's energy.

Cooking did more than just enable profound physiological changes in the human body and brain. It ignited sociality.[8] According to the contemporary British archeobotanist Martin Jones, the hearth certainly inspired sharing food, or what is now called commensality. The hearth also sparked sharing stories and fueled technological innovations for preparing, cooking, and consuming food.[9] Our ancestors flourished the more they integrated flames and food.

Human civilization was off and cooking.

Fire played a significant role in material technology as well. In his masterful 1973 history of science, *The Ascent of Man*, British historian of science Jacob Bronowski highlights many of the ways humans used fire to take matter apart and forge new material, particularly metal. Flames, in essence, functioned as a dynamic knife.

Physical knives had long played a central role for humankind. Sharp material objects enabled our ancestors to chop large foodstuffs into bite-size and even smaller pieces, which facilitated easier and quicker consumption, especially in precarious environs. We continue to use knives for this reason to this day. Knives are a way to outsource our metabolism: they do the work our teeth would otherwise need to do. With knives, our hands masticate the world. This intimate relationship between knives and food is captured in a rabbinic midrash: "Why is the knife called [in Hebrew] *ma'akhelet*? Because it makes food [*akilot*] fit to be eaten."[10] Since they share the same Hebrew root, *knives* and *food* are as etymologically related as they are phenomenologically vital to human survival.

Knives cut things we can see; fire cuts what we cannot. In Bronowski's words, "Physics is the knife that cuts into the grain of nature; fire, the flaming sword, is the kind that cuts below the visible structure, into the stone."[11] Through time and in all terrains, humans endeavored to master fire and develop myriad ways to cut food with blade and flame.

Other mammals, by contrast, continued their raw diets, be it vegetarian or carnivorous or omnivorous. These uncooked diets had morphological consequences. Since noncooking (and noncutting) vegetarians must always forage their food and masticate for hours to smash it into reasonably digestible bits, their jaws and bellies are massive. From beginning to end, their digestive tracts require immense levels of energy.

Carnivores, by contrast, sport slimmer guts so they can more easily chase prey, as depicted in a sketch by the nineteenth-century British natural history artist Benjamin Waterhouse Hawkins. Though each bite of flesh may contain more calories and protein than a random vegetarian mouthful, digesting flesh nonetheless burdens the body, requiring much energy and time, so carnivorous creatures often eat less frequently than vegetarian ones.

We cooking and cutting omnivores have a dramatically different morphology than our fellow mammals. Our bodies (can) carry a comparatively small paunch because of the ways in which we prepare our foods. Since we have outsourced many aspects of digestion to cooking,

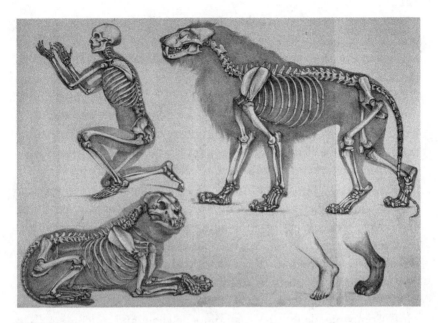

FIGURE 9.2

Benjamin Waterhouse Hawkins, "A Comparative View of the Human and Animal Frame,"
1860. *Wikimedia Commons.* https://commons.wikimedia.org/wiki/File:Comparative
_view_of_the_human_and_lion_frame,_Benjamin_Waterhouse_Hawkins,_1860.jpg.

our bodies need not work as hard as other vegetarian and carnivorous
mammals' nor bulk up as a consequence of that work. Our relatively slim
waists, compared to those of our genetic neighbors whose diets remain
raw, reflect the fact that our complex and cooked diets enable significant
proportions of the eaten energy to be diverted away from the digestive
tract itself to our gray matter. With less grinding to do, our teeth also
shrank, allowing our jaws to recalibrate bone and muscle into our current
physiological structure.

Cooking proved ingenious: it made us thinner *and* smarter. More,
cooking helped us stay healthy by detoxifying food. In short, cooking
proved to be an evolutionarily adaptive consumptive strategy.

Even if these reasons had been enough to keep cooking, our ancestors
(and we today) also wanted to continue cooking because it elicited incredible smells and, consequently, wonderful tastes. Searing flesh, boiling

broths, sautéing vegetables, baking breads, and brewing coffee—cooking produced smells so delicious we drooled like Pavlov's dogs. Why? What is it about cooked meat and crusty bread and aromatic coffee that so pleases and entices us?

We can thank the fin de siècle French physician and chemist Louis-Camille Maillard, who, after studying kidney diseases, became fascinated with the reactions between amino acids and sugars. In 1912 he noticed that these elements combine to create new odors, colors, and flavors when submitted to high heat: they become the bread's brown crust, the meat's crispy skin. Heat caused these acids and sugars to produce volatile and complex molecules, mixtures we find odorously beguiling and intensely delicious. This browning process, now called the Maillard reaction, is critical for those who cook to eat. It tells us when something is ready for consumption. The modern food industry deploys the Maillard reaction to stimulate us to buy certain foodstuffs. Just walk by a bread or donut shop, a fried chicken vender, or a coffee stand and take a whiff. Companies deliberately waft those delicious and enticing smells to cause us to drool, come in, and purchase a taste or two. Cooking thus uses and takes advantage of our biological sense of smell.

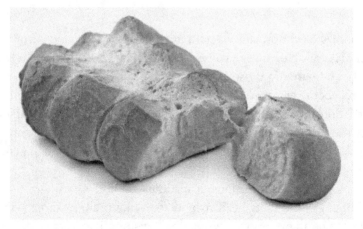

**FIGURE 9.3**

The delicious-smelling brown crust of bread is an example of the Maillard reaction.

Given the biological importance of cooking to our very existence and evolution, perhaps our species should be renamed *Homo gastronomicus*, the genus that cooks. Few other species go to the lengths we do to prepare meals. We are the only species that cooks food.[12]

Cooking may be our singular distinctive feature relative to Earth's other denizens, but perhaps we should hesitate before abandoning our current scientific moniker. The species of great apes—*Homo sapiens*—is so named because the Latin *sapere* means "to be wise." We anointed ourselves with this name because on the whole we admire wisdom and the large brain in our heads.

Yet are our wisdom and large brains truly what distinguishes us from all other creatures? Are these heady features what make us a unique species?

Recent work in animal studies reveals that the human brain is not the largest or even the most sophisticated out there; other mammals, like cetaceans and elephants, and certain primates also have substantial and variegated brains relative to their body size.[13] Further, many other species exist in exquisite harmony with each other and their neighbors, not just flourishing but living with wisdom, even ethicality.[14]

Though humans are not the sole proprietors of big brains or wisdom, we nonetheless can salvage the label *Homo sapiens*. Another meaning of *sapere* is "to taste" or "to have taste" (e.g., *sapid* means "savory"). Surely the wise have taste. *Homo sapiens* is the species of ape that tastes and has (good) taste.

Of course, this does not mean other species do not taste. Nor does it imply that other species do not have standards by which they measure each other and the world, standards akin to what we might call taste or moral sensibility. Rather, our scientific name reflects and reinforces the fact that tasting is what makes us us. We are the ones who savor.

On this point, Serres describes humankind as having two mouths.[15] The first mouth is first not because it came first but because it predominates and distracts; it is the mouth that speaks out into the world. The other is the mouth that brings the world within; it is the consuming and tasting mouth. As noted earlier, Serres holds that wisdom is subsequent to taste: "Knowledge cannot come to those who have neither tasted nor smelled. Speaking is not sapience, the first tongue needs the second. We were too quick to forget that *homo sapiens* refers to those who react to sapidity, appreciate it and seek it out, those for whom the sense of taste matters—savouring animals—before referring to judgment, intelligence or wisdom, before referring to talking man."[16] We are savoring animals before we can be sagacious. The words we use to describe the world come from our bodily encounter with it, particularly, if not primarily, from our consumption of it.

Savoring certainly involves the biological processes of bringing food and drink into the mouth, of smelling scents and odors, and mingling those with mouthfeel sensations like temperature and texture. It also requires the brain to integrate these senses into a fulsome experience, what is now known as the flavor experience. All that is tasting.

But savoring is something a bit more sophisticated than merely tasting the world. An activity of the mind, to savor is to reflect upon the tasting experience. More, it is to enjoy the tasting experience; it is to relish. Perhaps we are the sole species that relishes and savors its food; we are *Homo sapiens* in the fullest sense of its Latin root. We are the species that tastes, savors, and (eventually) expounds wisdom.

Both the synesthetic or multimodal nature of tasting and the mental dimensions of savoring inform our unique way of consuming the world-not-us.

We should pause for a moment to recall that nearly two centuries ago Brillat-Savarin admitted he was "tempted to believe that smell and taste form a single sense, of which the mouth is the laboratory and the nose is the chimney; or, to speak more exactly, of which one serves for the tasting of actual bodies and the other for the savoring of their gases."[17] He was not alone in considering taste and smell a singular sensation; Kant, too, held this opinion.[18] Brillat-Savarin nevertheless distinguished three sequential sensations in tasting. First, the direct sensation we feel is when food sits on the fore part of the tongue. Second, the complete sensation adds to the first "the impression which arises when the food leaves its original position, passes to the back of the mouth, and attacks the whole organ with its taste and its aroma." Third, the reflection sensation is "the opinion which one's spirit forms from the impressions which have been transmitted to it by the mouth."[19] Three locales (mouth, nose, brain) and three interconnected experiences (taste, aroma, reflection) constitute tasting in its fullest. They constitute savoring.

For this reason, connoisseurs hesitate. Gourmands take time between sips and nibbles to appreciate fully the beauty of both what they are eating and the eating experience itself. Is there any surprise, then, that Brillat-Savarin insists that tasting and savoring are the sense and experience that give us the greatest joy?

Long before the pleasing dainties of nineteenth-century France, maybe as long as three thousand years ago in what is now northern India, Brahmins compiled the *Upanishads*, collections of Vedic philosophies and instructions from which Hinduism and Buddhism emerged. This ancient source speaks of the fivefold constitution of the human self, which is the accumulative and sequential integration of food, breath, mind, intelligence, and bliss.[20] Given what we now know about the physiology of taste, this ordering is uncannily prescient. Humans have long known, then, that when food and air mingle in our minds, wisdom builds and great happiness becomes possible.

To savor is to be happily human.

## A TASTY TRINITY

*Quod sapid nutrit*—What is tasteful is nutritious—is an aphorism supposedly coined by Abū ʿAlī al-Ḥusayn ibn ʿAbd Allāh ibn Al-Hasan ibn Ali ibn Sīnā, known as Avicenna, the great eleventh-century Persian philosopher of medicine and science.[21] How lovely were this true. The "tasty" are unequally nutritious, however.

Some tastes are more equal than others, more intense, more desired. Others are neutral, some avoided, and still others are considered disgusting. Over the millennia, however, three tastes, or macronutrients, have emerged as particularly sought after. Indeed, their attractiveness is so intense that the modern Westernized industrial food complex, if we may reasonably speak of it in homogeneous terms, structures itself more or less around these three. The ubiquity of these three tastes often goes unnoticed until it is pointed out that their increasing prevalence in recent decades maps nearly in correlation with society's ballooning weight issues and correlated health problems.

What are these delicious yet perhaps nefarious tastes? Are they really only deleterious to our health? Should we consider them forbidden fruits and never consume them despite our desire for them? Or may we continue to enjoy them?

Go ahead, refrain . . . or never indulge in the first place? What might an adaptive consumptive strategy be for this tasty trinity?

Many sciences today identify sugar, fat, and salt as central contributors to our ever-expanding waistlines and faltering health. For a variety of reasons, we eagerly consume these three ingredients, frequently and in great quantities. Nearly every meal and snack and many drinks we ingest have them in abundance. Avoiding them is hard, especially in the modern food environment in which most of us live and eat. Yet as our bodies progressively show, our desire for them has morbid and even mortal consequences for us.

But we should not jump to the conclusion that we ought never to consume them. On the contrary. We need sugar, fat, and salt to exist.

Without carbohydrates, lipids, and salts, our bodies fail and die. No civilization or culinary culture has ever existed that did not rely upon these ingredients to some degree. Nor has any individual human ever survived for long without any one of them.

Though dangerous, these ingredients are nonetheless vital. Place this fact in conversation with Derrida's urgent question: Since we must eat salt, sugar, and fat, how can we eat them well?

To answer this question, we need to appreciate how these ingredients are both dangerous and enlivening. Some people would rather pass by these details in favor of figuring out how much of these ingredients we should eat. Theirs is the impulse to pursue an idealized solution. For example, some authorities, like the U.S. government's recommended daily allowance (RDA), suggest the answer is a precise quantity: all of us should eat only so much salt and so many fats. (Though the American Heart Association nonetheless suggests all adult men should consume no more than 9 teaspoons of added sugar per day and adult women 6 teaspoons, the powerful sugar lobby continues to prevent the government from declaring an advisement on the amount of sugar to consume per day. That is why there is no official RDA for sugar.) This model assumes people have the wherewithal, time, and focus to measure everything we put into our mouths.

At the other extreme, some authors and authorities urge us to avoid one or another ingredient altogether. There is no need to slow down and measure our consumption of fat, say, because it should not be eaten at all. By ruling out a particular ingredient, these authors work with the presumption that we get enough of the ingredient in a particular prescribed diet regimen that, surprise, surprise, is the very one they propose.

Such approaches do little to advance our overall understanding of how and why these three ingredients are simultaneously vital and lethal. These one-size-fits-all panaceas may not be panaceas at all, in part because no two bodies are exactly alike. Since my body differs from yours, the amount of sugar, fat, and salt I need to live well will not and probably should not be the same as what you need to consume. And as I grow, develop, mature, and senesce, my body's metabolic needs necessarily change. A prescriptive regimen for a population thus cannot be adequate for all its individual members in all stages of their lives.

Now, to be fair, expecting generalized programs like the RDA to be sensitive to the unique needs of each individual body would be an unreasonable requirement. Equally, leaving individuals to figure out ideal consumption levels of these particular macronutrients would be an unnecessary burden. Given how enticing fat, sugar, and salt are, free rein could be a recipe for personal and collective disaster.

A more nuanced approach would be wiser, specifically, an approach that understands each person as a unique consumer with idiosyncratic metabolic needs and hedonic interests. We need an approach that educates and motivates each person to consume according not to external cues (e.g., RDAs or the like) as much as by internal cues. Eating well requires each person to eat enough, or just right, of these three ingredients.

## NECESSARY CRAVINGS

Since we must eat salt, sugar, and fat, why do we crave them beyond what is otherwise healthy for us?

Recall *Homo gastronomicus*: cooking sparked human brain growth, made us more svelte, freed great swaths of our time from foraging so we could pursue other adventures and ideas, and dramatically altered our social lives. Cooking makes us us, and cooking makes us nearly uncontrollably eager for salts, sugars, and fats.

Cooking and craving go hand in hand.

Consider the barbecue. Indisputably the oldest way we heated food, cooking over flames creates mesmerizing and salivating sights, sounds, smells, temperatures, textures, and tastes. Something about this kind of cooking attracts us.

Maillard's discovery is key here. He realized that under the pressure of heat amino acids combine with carbohydrates (which need not be only sugars) to create new and volatile tastants (molecules our tongues sense) and flavors (smells our noses add to those tastes). The Maillard reaction may be a new name for it, but this technique to make our foods even more enticing is age-old. We use the Maillard reaction ubiquitously today in nearly every corner of the food industry. Caramelization is another, similar transformation heat produces in foods. Here, sugars or carbohydrates (but not amino acids) undergo permanent chemical restructuring. These derivative chemicals are not just nuttier and sweeter than the original raw ingredients; they are all the more delicious.

As Michael Pollan, the contemporary American food journalist, describes in his book *Cooked*, barbecues and any cooking over fire generally does this food transformation par excellence.[22] These new textures, colors, sounds, tastes, smells, and flavors brought about by fire's high heat excite us in part precisely because they do not exist in nature. Flame cooking—all cooking, for that matter—adds fresh dimensions to food that cannot be produced by raw foods, no matter the recipe. No wonder, then, that we have long loved food fresh off the grill or out of the oven. But our love for cooked foods is not just because they produce wonderful flavors. We seek them because we need them.

Again, the elements transformed so enticingly in many cooking processes are amino acids and carbohydrates. Our bodies need both. We need amino acids because they enable the body's cells to perform proper protein synthesis. Inadequate consumption of amino acids causes enervating physical and neurological reactions: nervousness, dizziness, and overall exhaustion. Essential amino acids are found in plants as well as animals. While animal proteins offer the most abundant source of these necessary amino acids, through millennia of experimentation civilizations around the world discovered combinations of plants that also provide sufficient amounts of complete proteins and the necessary amino acids, such as corn and beans or soybeans and rice. Humans thus do not need to consume meat; we need the essential amino acids contained in meats and in certain vegetarian combinations.

Our bodies need carbohydrates, too. When metabolized, they produce sugars like glucose that provide short-term energy. Sweet foods and drinks shortcut this process by providing glucose and other sugars directly to our guts. Glucose in our blood stimulates insulin, the hormone responsible for metabolizing glucose. When functioning properly, insulin causes liver cells, muscles, and fat tissues to absorb excess sugar from the blood lest its concentration there become toxic. Muscles then utilize the sugars to do what we bid them to do. If sugar levels fall too low, the hormone glucagon that is produced by the pancreas causes the liver to convert and release its stored glucose into the bloodstream. These and other peptide, or digestive, hormones keep blood sugar levels within healthy limits. As discussed in chapter 5, this is homeostasis, a self-regulating system. So what happens if we do not utilize all the sugar's energy that we have consumed? Extra sugars not immediately used by the body are transformed through a process called fatty acid synthesis, and these eventually become fat repositories of stored energy the body can transform back into usable sugars if and when they are needed. In brief, unused sugars become adipose tissue or fat deposits, bulking up our frames and becoming baggage we must cart around wherever we go.

That we crave what we bodily need makes great sense. For us not to crave such biological necessities would be evolutionarily disadvantageous. In this instance, we should be thankful that our wants match our needs. We love to barbecue vegetables no less than meats precisely because our bodies can get from this kind of cooking both essential amino acids and critical carbs. We salivate in anticipation for what salves—and saves—us.

Our bodies have another elemental need, salt, whose ions—sodium and chloride—are vital for all living organisms. Together they help control the fluid balance (volume, pH, and blood pressure) in an organism. Regulated in humans by the kidneys, chloride is needed for metabolism and sodium is needed for our nervous system's electrical signaling. Potassium chloride is another salt whose elements are similarly vital for our body's functions. Too much of a salt in our system can cause morbid ailments like high blood pressure and mortal outcomes from strokes and cardiovascular diseases. At the other extreme, too little salt can lead to electrolyte disturbances, dizziness, and even death.

Ironically, salt is so necessary for human flourishing that it has been the cause of a great many conflicts. Wars have been fought to gain access to and control of saline sources. Just as the singular organic body cannot survive without an adequate supply of salt, cities, empires, and whole civilizations must also have steady sources of salt to avoid economic and political destabilization. A strong relationship between despotic governments and salt revenues was first observed in the 1875 book, *Das Salz*, written by the German romantic naturalist Matthias J. Schleiden, who helped develop cell theory, the theory that all plants have cells. A century before him, in 1787, J. F. Barandiéry Montmayuer, the Count of Essuile, presciently warned that if the king wanted to preserve the saltworks in France, he would need to limit his taxation on salt. A few years later this very salt tax would be a contentious issue in the emerging French Revolution. In antiquity, the government's monopolistic control of salt was more than a financial scheme: salt was the medium of pay. In Roman times, for example, people were given "their worth in salt," that is, their salary. Governmental control over salt or the severe taxation of it to finance militaries was a longtime practice in China, with evidence going back some four thousand years.[23]

Though no blood was let, perhaps the most famous conflict over salt occurred in 1930 in India. With seventy-nine collaborators, the nonviolent independence activist Mohandas K. Gandhi set off from his ashram on the Sabarmati River in Ahmedabad on a month-long march south, covering some two hundred miles, to the Arabian Sea. Their goal: to demonstrate the injustice of Britain's monopolistic hold on India's salt. The drama of the march was unmistakable geopolitical theater. With waves crashing behind him, Gandhi, a slight man wearing just a thin dhoti and sandals, would bend down on the Dandi beach and pick up a hand of sandy sea salt and in so doing thwart the world's greatest empire and thereby gesture toward its ultimate crash into history. That simple grasp of naturally occurring sodium chloride rattled the world's most sophisticated global hegemony. Salt was the lifeblood of India, politically as well as biologically.

Since neither our political nor our personal bodies can spontaneously produce sufficient amino acids, glucose, or salt, we must consume them from the world around us. This existential fact reinforces the observations made earlier: we are imperfect beings unquestionably and radically dependent on consuming our environment. We must draw sustenance from outside ourselves and bring it in if we are to live at all. We must eat the world-not-us to be us.

But we must be careful when consuming these macroingredients. We risk injury and death if we abstain from these three critical ingredients altogether. At the other extreme, when we consume them with abandon, their abundance in our bodies also promises only trouble. Given that we are biologically oriented to crave these tasty ingredients, and given that eating too much of them would be as dangerous and maladaptive as eating too little of them, our challenge is to eat just enough of them to ensure our vitality. Of course, that amount is unique to each eater.

## THE BEAUTY OF TASTE

Another reason taste is so important to reflect upon is its very centrality to the ways we think and speak about the world. According to Australian scholar Elsbeth Probyn, "Taste distinguishes in an essential way, since taste is the basis of all that one has—people and things—and all that one is for others, whereby one classifies oneself and is classified by others."[24] Because taste is the very process by which we assess the world and ourselves interacting with that world, we differentiate the savory from the unsavory. Since each of us uses taste to make fine distinctions, taste becomes the language by which we articulate our approval and disapproval. Taste thus transcends our biological tongues by expressing notions of pleasure, agreeableness, and beauty. Through centuries of philosophical meditation, taste became "a suitable analog for judgments of the quality of experience by means of immediate, subjective approval."[25] Starting perhaps as early as the fifteenth century and certainly by the eighteenth,

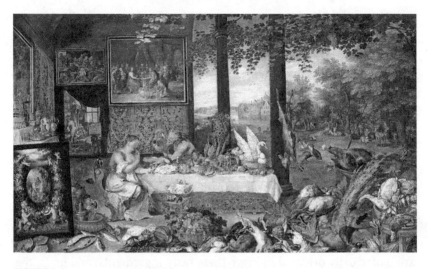

**FIGURE 9.4**

Jan Brueghel the Elder and Peter Paul Rubens, *Allegory of Taste*, 1618.

taste became bound up in if not the language for the field of knowledge we call aesthetics.

In a famous collaboration in early seventeenth-century Antwerp, Peter Paul Rubens and Jan Brueghel the Elder devised a series of five paintings depicting the basic senses: Rubens drew the figures while Brueghel completed the settings. For the sense of taste, they situated a woman at a banquet table overflowing with sumptuous foods, predominantly game. Piled around her are all sorts of fish, other sea creatures, fowl, land animals, fruits, and vegetables, while off in the distance animals meander undisturbed by the fleshy fare in the foreground. By her knee sits a massive bowl of fried and baked sweets,[26] while behind her a multitiered buffet has myriad carafes and more delicacies. More impressive than the sheer quantity of food and drink are the several bird pies elegantly arranged on the white tablecloth. These sumptuous items "would have expressed to an early modern viewer the wealth of a household that could afford to possess and staff a large oven and other baking technologies required."[27] Indeed, the kitchen, hidden behind a drape momentarily drawn up, reveals laborers, even more raw foods, and such cooking technologies as a chopping block and hatchet, a hearth with rotisserie, skewers, and more. The relative calm in this kitchen inverts the chaos of the one depicted in the painting above the doorway—*The Fat Kitchen* by Pieter van der Heyden that we studied in chapter 2.

Even as these surroundings imbue this consumptive moment with great economic import and sensory delight, our attention is drawn to the painting's center, where the lady brings a morsel (probably an oyster) to her mouth. A crouching tamarin monkey gnaws on its own food behind her while a satyr in front of her plies her with even more wine. Hardly delighting in the real and mythological bounty surrounding her, indifferent to their temptations and vices, she sups as if alone.

However much we, the observers, might want to be precisely where she is, tasting that incredible array of dishes in that particular setting, we are not and cannot sit in her stead. Only she is there, and she alone is the one who can enjoy—or not—the fare. She is the final and only judge of whether what she tastes is indeed tasty.

Taste, whether it be of food or surroundings, is ultimately idiosyncratic.[28]

Yet taste is also profoundly social.

Calling someone insipid is to insult that person. On one level, *insipid* means "to be without taste or perceptible flavor," whereas on another it means "tasteless, uninteresting, dull, boring." To be insipid is to be uninteresting, uninspiring. (The word is also linked with *jejune*, meaning "dull in the mind, flat, wanting in interest," itself a word linked with the digestive tract.) As the contemporary British novelist Julian Barnes observes, "We may be better or worse people, happy or miserable, successful or failing, but what we *are*, within these wider categories, how we define ourselves, as opposed to how we are genetically defined, is what we call 'taste.' Yet the word—perhaps because of its broad catchment area—easily misleads. 'Taste' can imply calm reflection; while its derivatives—tasteful, tastefulness, tasteless, tastelessness—lead us into a world of minute differentiations, of snobbery, social values and soft furnishings."[29] One's taste indicates one's sociability. A tasteless person is insensitive to others, invasive of others' privacy, hoarding for personal hedonistic pleasures, and ultimately indifferent to others' needs and interests. We call that person not merely insipid but distasteful. Similarly, a tasteless society lacks solidarity, cohesion, and companionship.

By contrast, a person of taste reflects upon or thinks about others because he or she realizes that individual consumption has communal implications. This creature who tastes the world (specifically salt, sugar, and fat) and has good taste (by thinking about and, as we shall see, caring for others) is none other than a *Homo sapiens*. The beauty of taste thus resides not just in its aesthetics but in its ethics, too.

# 10

## SACRIFICING

*One's eating is thought to be a perfect act of worship
like one of the forms of divine service.*

—Bahya ben Asher ibn Halawa, *Shulḥan Shel Arba* (1514)

Strong biological reasons exist for us to crave sweets, fats, and salts. We can hardly survive without them, yet at the other extreme, we can hardly survive when we gorge on them. Our culinary ingenuity complicates matters further. Cooking transforms these macronutrients so they become nearly irresistible. Restraining ourselves from consuming these necessities without being excessive is more than a question of vital importance. It is one of theological significance.

Even as they acknowledge our hankering for sweets, fats, and salts, several religious traditions—Judaism, Christianity, and Islam in particular—adamantly warn against devouring them without restraint. To do so would be theologically impertinent. On the other hand, these traditions do not teach that we are completely forbidden from eating these mouthwatering ingredients. Rather, we are to constrain our consumption of them. Though we may taste them, we should eat less of them than we otherwise could or want to.

Go ahead, refrain.

Before we can even contemplate restraining ourselves from eating some of the tastiest things in this flavorful world, let us consider when, according to these traditions, tasty foods came into being in the first place.

In the first creation story humans are given seed-bearing trees and seed-bearing fruit to eat. No other words are given to describe this fare. The trees in the Garden of Eden in the second creation story are much more interesting, gustatorily speaking. God plants in that garden nutritious trees, aesthetically pleasing trees, and peculiar trees. The tree of moral knowledge that Eve considers is simultaneously "good for eating, a delight to the eyes, and a desirable source of wisdom."[1] Might this mean that moral knowledge tastes good?

Perhaps. Or maybe this tree's enticement links to Eve's and Adam's very being. Whereas in the first creation story humans are fashioned in God's image and have no explicit material corpora, in this second version they are formed out of dust and divine breath. As biological creatures who must breathe to exist, Eve and Adam can taste as well. Appealing to their sense of taste thus makes sense. This theological theory of human ontology corroborates what we have learned from science. We organic creatures must breathe to be and to taste.[2]

The third creation story adds a fascinating wrinkle to this theology of being, breathing, and tasting. Immediately upon disembarking from the ark Noah offers clean animals and birds to God upon a flaming altar. This primordial fiery sacrifice produces pleasing smells for God, and their scent inspires God to commit to never again annihilate all living things on account of humankind.[3] God can breathe in the smells of this world only because Noah acted on an impulse to offer a sacrifice in the first place. The significance of this idea is immense. Noah's was a primal gesture of offering over (and up) to the divine Other what he himself could have consumed. Instead of eating this tasty, fleshy, and fiery fare, he gave it away. Tasting and smelling the world inextricably intertwine with sacrificing.

Weaving together these foundational stories we can see that to taste the world well involves giving some of it away. To taste well—to eat well—involves consuming some but less than what one otherwise could ingest.

## SWEETS

Consider sweets. In the ancient Levantine world on the eastern side of the Mediterranean Ocean in which Judaism, Christianity, and eventually Islam emerged, honey and dates were two of the sweetest ingredients around. Sugarcane, by contrast, was first cultivated in Papau New Guinea around 10,000 years ago and introduced into the region by Arabs

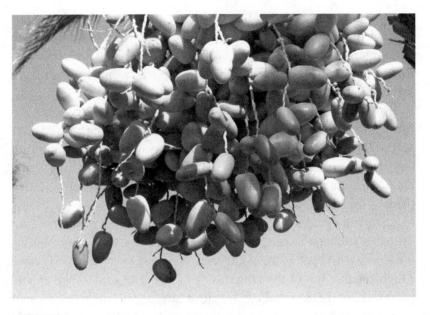

**FIGURE 10.1**

The common date has long been a source of sugar and other nutrients throughout the Mediterranean Basin.

only about 1,400 to 1,300 years ago. Most of the religious teachings, including those within Islam, thus refer to naturally occurring sweeteners involving dates and honey and not to crystalized sugar.

What is curious is that these religious traditions maintain ambivalence toward these saccharine wonders. This ambivalence is perhaps clearest in the Jewish textual tradition. The early rabbis recognized that extreme hunger demands the quick acquisition of calories, though of course they knew nothing of calories as such. They taught, "If someone is seized by ravenous hunger, feed him honey and all sorts of sweets, for they enlighten the eyes of man."[4] This simple teaching seems straightforward at first flush: the rabbis think consuming naturally occurring sugar is a good way to rejuvenate the extremely famished. However, the context of this source suggests otherwise. This piece of advice is found in a larger discussion about choosing between options, and specifically about ranking the less bad, or the less forbidden, of two options. For instance, feeding someone carrion (animals whose cause of death is unknown) is less bad than giving a person food that has not been properly tithed. This larger context thus gives greater precision to the rabbinic teaching: feeding sweets to the famished may be allowable, but it is not commended unconditionally.

This somewhat conservative attitude toward consuming sweets has roots in the biblical story of Jonathan and his father, King Saul.[5] At war against the Philistines, Saul ordered his military not to eat anything until their gruesome tasks were done. Fearing the gravity of their king's oath, his soldiers ate none of the abundant honey that dripped down around them to the forest floor. At this time Jonathan was ahead of the troops, scouting and slaughtering foes; so far ahead was he that he did not hear his father's ban on sweets. When he saw the abundant honey, he took some, raised his hand to his mouth, and, upon tasting it, "his eyes became enlightened."[6] One of the king's soldiers was with him, however, and informed him of the royal curse against anyone who ate this honey, or anything else for that matter. Jonathan wondered why his father would hamstring his own troops, for had they been nourished on food, or at least on this bounteous honey, their successes against the Philistines would have been even greater.

The ambivalence is unmistakable. Given that honey is a potent invigorator, the government assumes the right, even the responsibility to regulate its consumption, especially during wartime.[7] Is it any surprise, then, that sugar was one of the first consumables to be rationed during World War II, starting in 1940 in the United Kingdom? In the United States, sugar was also the first item curtailed, as explained in the *War Ration Book Number One*, distributed in May 1942, also known as "The Sugar Book."

Even if individuals were free to eat sweets during times of relative peace, ancient proverbs warned against guzzling them. For example:

"If you find honey, eat only what you need, lest, surfeiting yourself, you
  throw it up."
"It is not good to eat a lot of honey."
"A sated person loathes honeycomb, but to a famished person everything
  bitter is sweet."[8]

Whoever penned such aphorisms was wary of sweets because they beguile the palate and confound the gut. Eating too much of them will have negative, expulsive consequences.

This guardedness toward sweets never diminished in Western civilization, or at least in certain segments of it. The Nation of Islam in twentieth-century America, for example, eschewed sweets. Elijah Muhammad, the leader who succeeded Master Fard Muhammad, repeatedly wrote in his two-volume *How to Eat to Live* that sweets were to be abjured because they only pollute the body, causing and exacerbating diabetes as well as a whole host of other physical if not psychological maladies.[9]

At the other extreme, however, is the famous depiction of the biblical Land of Israel as "flowing with milk and honey."[10] As enticing and bucolic as this vision may be, milk and honey are not produced by the land gratis: they require labor. Securing a regular source of milk involves intensive husbanding of ruminant herds of cows, goats, or sheep. Extracting honey requires beekeepers risking injury and even death every time they go near hives. So while milk and honey may be delicious, they come at a cost of labor, calories, and sometimes even life itself.

Ambivalence toward sweet things is also found in Christianity. When the Apostle John is bidden to eat a scroll that was held in an angel's hands, he learns that sweet-tasting things can sour stomachs.[11] This little story contains a huge theological contention. It points to an old and strongly held conviction connecting sweets and God. Earlier the Hebrew Bible teaches that sweet-smelling incense is meant for God's olfactory pleasure and not for human stimulation.[12] Indeed, it was this sweet smell that first inspired God to promise never to destroy the world again.[13] (The practice of offering up sweet incense for divine pleasure is as commonplace today in India as it has ever been.) Metaphorically, too, there is a link between God and sweets. About God's judgments and teachings King David sang, "They are more desirable than gold, even fine gold, sweeter than honey and the honeycomb" and "How sweet are your words to my palate, sweeter than honey in my mouth."[14] Perhaps the divine scroll John ingests is too sweet for his biological constitution (thus causing his indigestion) but just right to stimulate his spiritual convictions.

Another way to appreciate John's experience is to remember that consuming sweet things is not bad in and of itself, but it can be dangerous if done improperly or with poor attention or wayward intentions.[15] The potency of sugar must be respected. Remember, too, sugars stimulate fermentation.

Humans have long observed that, when given the right circumstances, naturally high-fructose fruits like dates and grapes ferment into powerful and palatable alcoholic concoctions. Imbibing too much of these alcoholic drinks can cause problems. Just ask Noah. His second impulse after disembarking from the ark in which he, his family, and all the world's animals had been cramped during the flood was to plant a vineyard. He may have been a skilled oenologist, but no teetotaler was he: he immediately got drunk, as is well known, and bad things ensued.[16] Sometimes sweet drinks produce bitter results.

Later, Moses reminds the Israelites that even in moderation, wine induces laxity if not rebellion.[17] The impulse to forewarn the masses against wanton consumption of fermented drinks became a theological pastime for Judaism, Christianity, and Islam.[18] That prophets and religions in general felt compelled to remind their constituents (again and again) to be careful with their alcoholic drinks suggests that their communities were in actuality not so careful. To combat such excessiveness, some traditions and strains within other traditions went so far as to outlaw the consumption of alcohol altogether (Islam, Mormonism, Jainism, Sikkhism, Baha'i, among others).

Even though unfermented sweets are from and even for God, it is unnecessary—theologically speaking—to avoid consuming them altogether. On the contrary, many religions insist that we should consume *some* sweets and alcohol. For example, in the fifth century BCE, the prophet Ezra instituted a new way to encounter revelation. He read the Hebrew Torah aloud in public and simultaneously translated it into the vernacular, Aramaic, making God's teaching intelligible to the crowd. Overcome, the people wept. Nehemiah, then the governor, implored the people not to cry but rather to celebrate: "Go, eat choice [fatty] food and drink sweet things, and send some to those who have nothing prepared, for this day is holy to our God."[19] How brilliant and revolutionary this is! Ezra's novel reading practice democratized divine wisdom; no longer should the literate elite control it. More, people were to link divine wisdom with earthly consumption, spiritual guidance with physical nourishment. The

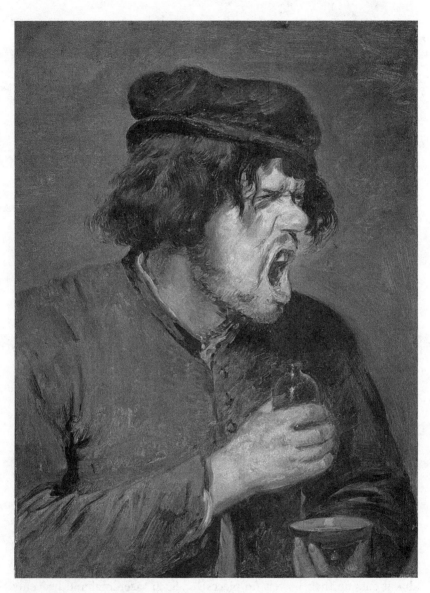

**FIGURE 10.2**

Adriean Brouwer, *The Bitter Draft*, 1636.

two go hand in hand, much as the rabbis would teach centuries later, "If there is no flour, there is no Torah; if no Torah, no flour."[20] And as Mohammad would teach regarding sweets, wisdom, and healing: "And from the fruit of the date-palm and the vine, ye get out wholesome drink and food: behold, in this also is a sign for those who are wise. And thy Lord taught the Bee to build its cells in hills, on trees, and in (men's) habitations; Then to eat of all the produce (of the earth), and find with skill the spacious paths of its Lord: there issues from within their bodies a drink of varying colours, wherein is healing for men: verily in this is a Sign for those who give thought,"[21] Note, too, the final gesture Nehemiah instituted: the people were to *share* their sweet drinks and choice food with those who had none. Wisdom and sweets are designed to be distributed, not hoarded.

Just as sweets are not to be eschewed altogether, the strong attitudes against indiscriminate consumption of fermented drinks are also not absolute. Legion are the instructions in the Torah and rabbinic literature about drinking wine before and during Jewish celebrations. Shabbat itself is to be properly opened and closed by blessing and drinking wine. In Christianity, wine has long been associated with Jesus's blood and consumed throughout the centuries by believers. Though Paul the Apostle taught Timothy that wine should be drunk to protect the body from ailments that arise from impure water, Paul stresses that only a little wine should be drunk.[22] The Qur'anic vision of heavenly rewards for true believers includes imbibing a wine so pure it causes no headache, only joy and bliss: "(Here is) a Parable of the Garden which the righteous are promised: in it are rivers of water incorruptible; rivers of milk of which the taste never changes; rivers of wine, a joy to those who drink; and rivers of honey pure and clear. In it there are for them all kinds of fruits; and Grace from their Lord. (Can those in such Bliss) be compared to such as shall dwell forever in the Fire, and be given, to drink, boiling water, so that it cuts up their bowels (to pieces)?"[23] Such sacerdotal and heavenly dimensions of wine echo and reinforce the idea shared across these traditions that not all sugars or their derivatives are inherently bad and should be avoided. Nor are these sweet items meant for unconstrained human consumption. On the contrary. All traditions imbue sweets and alcohol with symbolic and theological powers. Go ahead, enjoy, and also refrain lest things go awry. Also, just as divine knowledge is to be distributed across the community, so sweets and wine are to be shared. Neither sacred knowledge nor sucrose is to be monopolized; the spiritually and physically ethical consumption of them requires otherwise.

## FATS

A similar story can be told about fat. While the biblical prohibition against eating blood is well known, the one against consuming fat has been all but forgotten.[24] The Levitical instructions of properly sacrificing animals are concise and clear: "All the fat is God's."[25] The fat surrounding and attached to the entrails, kidneys, and liver are not to be consumed except by the altar's fire. In addition to forbidding the population from eating such fats from butchered animals, even the fat of animals who died naturally or by other beasts is prohibited. The consequence was severe: anyone who eats those fats must be cut off from the community.[26] Anyone consuming animal blood also must be excised from the community. Why, though, are humans forbidden from consuming blood and fat?

The blood prohibition has a clear biblical rationale. No less than God explains it to Noah: blood is the stuff of life, and spilling it merits a reckoning.[27]

However, no clear reason exists in the Bible for the proscription against consuming fat. Contemporary American scholar of religion Susan Hill offers possible interpretations in *Eating to Excess: The Meaning of Gluttony and the Fat Body in the Ancient World*. For example, fat—suet, really, as muscle tissue always contains some fat—represents either deep-seated human emotions, the best of which are to be devoted to God, or perhaps aspects of human nature God detests and thus wants immolated. Fat is to be admired or abjured.

A tighter understanding of the fat prohibition derives from the other kinds of sacrifices among which it is listed.[28] Those other sacrifices are to be from one's best possessions—the best grains, the purest animals. All these best things are to be given over to God. Hill reasons that fat, too, must be "the best" both nutritionally and symbolically. Indeed, many cultures view suet or blubber not just as a delicacy but as a necessary ingredient for survival. Yet whereas the blood prohibition "stands as a warning to humans to be mindful of the sacredness of life, the prohibition against eating fat stands as a warning to humans about the dangers of excess."[29] We saw a glimpse of this when Moses linked the consumption of sweets and fatty foods to collective recalcitrance. On his view, eating beyond what is divinely permitted fuels idolatry.[30]

We can make this interpretation about fat even clearer. Whereas fat in permitted animal flesh is unavoidable because it is inseparable from the muscle in which it is found, the fat earmarked for God is clearly identifiable and separable. Visceral fat can be easily identified within the body cavity and carefully removed from those portions permitted for consumption. Choosing to eat animal flesh (remember, eating meat is a concession, not a requirement, for humankind) must involve distinguishing appropriate from inappropriate fats. This choice requires giving away—specifically to God—the very best fats and eating less than what one might otherwise.

The call not to eat all fats carries on in Christianity. Though the Christian Bible says little about consuming fat per se, Paul expresses an early attitude about eating meat. He calls upon true believers to refrain from passing judgment on others who divide all food and meat in particular into clean and unclean categories. Not only that, if one's eating habits offend others, one should adjust what one eats and how, lest one cause others to stumble.[31] This practice has profound potency, Paul claims. Such voluntary consumptive self-restraint by believers enriches social relations as much as it protects God's kingdom from unnecessary destruction: "For the kingdom of God is not food and drink but righteousness and peace and joy in the Holy Spirit. The one who thus serves Christ is acceptable to God and has human approval. Let us then pursue what makes for peace and for mutual upbuilding. Do not, for the sake of food, destroy the work of God. Everything is indeed clean, but it is wrong for you to make others fall by what you eat; it is good not to eat meat or drink wine or do anything that makes your brother or sister stumble."[32] Eating—and eating meat in particular—can mend or rend human society and God's kingdom. Though it may not be a central tenet in many streams of current Christianity, early Christianity acknowledges eating's social and theological power.

Connections between human consumption of fat and God's will and wisdom are also found in rabbinic literature. Early medieval rabbis wrote a parable about the verse "for in much wisdom is much vexation": "Two men entered a shop. One ate coarse bread and vegetables, while the other ate fine bread and fat meat, and drank old wine and partook of an oily sauce and came out feeling ill. The man who had 'fine food' suffered harm, while he who had 'coarse food' escaped harm."[33] The context of this parable in the midrash refers to study and the acquisition of divine knowledge, favorite pastimes of the rabbis. To wit, those who partake of sophisticated texts necessarily suffer the difficulty of absorbing them; they suffer more than those who content themselves with simple fare and base lessons. In this perhaps perverse way, intellectuals, the idealized gourmands of ideas and theology in that rabbinic world, were praised for their difficult labors. Rabbi Bahya disagrees with this teaching. For him, "fine foods" actually refine the intellect and make the heart clear-sighted, whereas "coarse foods" cloud the intellect and ruin both lucidity and refinement.[34]

Rabbi Bahya explores at length the interconnections among fats, class, and consumption in his *Shulḥan Shel Arba*, or *The Table of Four* (legs). Regarding the Talmudic teaching "An *'am ha'aretz* [commoner] may not eat the flesh of cattle, for it is said, *This is the law [Torah] of the beast, and of the fowl* (Leviticus 11:46); whoever engages in [the study of] the Torah may eat the flesh of beast and fowl, but he who does not engage in [the study of] the Torah may not eat the flesh of beast and fowl,"[35] Rabbi Bahya opines that nonscholars lack "intellectual souls" necessary to study sacred texts with fervor or understanding. They also lack the bodily wherewithal to eat meat and its fat. In his view, scholars have the illumination or intellectual fire to consume meat and its fat.[36] Their bellies have the necessary "fire" to consume denser, and more dangerous, fare. For contemporary professor of religion Jonathan Brumberg-Kraus, this passage means the individual scholar serves as both physical and metaphysical altar and fire upon which intellectual and meaty sacrifices are placed and consumed.[37]

Not all medievalists agree that eating meat should be permissible only to certain classes. One dissenter is Maimonides, the great twelfth-century physician and sage in Fostat, Egypt. He writes this to the Muslim vizier:

"All that is in the abdomen [of an animal] is bad. . . . [Such] Fat is all bad; it surfeits, corrupts the digestion."[38] In his more medical view, avoiding and regulating abdominal fat or suet is not done for symbolic theological or sociological purposes only. No one should ever consume suet because it has discomforting physiological consequences.

Maimonides's distaste for suet may have been strong, but it did not inspire him to prescribe a vegetarian, much less a vegan diet. In his writings we find several recommendations to eat small game and fowl. It seems his proscription against suet refers to the fats that can be easily separated out from an animal's carcass and muscle, much like the abdominal fats or suet identified in the Levitical sacrificial instructions. Go ahead and eat the fat internal to the muscles permitted for consumption, but refrain from eating those separable fats earmarked for God.

Though Islam permits the consumption of certain meats, fat itself is not on the menu. According to a hadith tradition, Mohammad once asked Umar, who was hosting him then, about the fat in the dish they were eating. Umar replied that he had searched in the market for bones with plenty of meat but they were too expensive. Instead he bought bones with little fat on them and added ghee, so that his family—and any guests he might have, like Mohammad himself—would go through the dish bone by bone. The hadith concludes with Umar noting that Mohammad never ate meat and milk together; he would eat one and give the other to charity.[39] While this hadith reinforces the Islamic tradition of not mixing dairy and meat, it also suggests that it is better to procure, cook, serve, and consume less fatty meats so to savor them all the more. A different hadith teaches that Mohammad was happiest when his Friday meal contained no fat.[40] Such teachings promote the idea that eating well requires limiting one's fat intake, perhaps even to nothing.

Given such enduring religious concerns about animal fats, should we be surprised that modern scientific studies of animal fats would endorse restricting their consumption? Suet provides incredible amounts of energy per volume unit, to be sure. Yet since it is nearly 100 percent fat, its protein content is negligible and its cholesterol is relatively high compared to many cuts of animal muscle.[41] Even more troubling is the finding that the fat of ruminant animals like cows and sheep contains 3 to 8 percent trans fats, perhaps the highest rate in naturally occurring foods, and these are the very fats implicated in coronary heart disease.[42] Though some recent studies are beginning to challenge the link between all trans fats and ill health, a scientific consensus remains: unless you are, say, an arctic explorer needing extra kilojoules of energy to survive in an extremely harsh environment, the biological return for eating suet and other rendered animal fat is not merely nil; it is dangerous.

Animal flesh and fat are not the only sources of trans fats in our modern diets. A more likely source comes from chemically hydrogenated polyunsaturated fats, especially vegetable oils. Because evidence accrues nearly daily of their deleterious effect on bodily health, efforts are being made throughout the contemporary food environment to curtail their use.

As with sweets, humans are theologically and biologically motivated to restrict their consumption of animal fats. People certainly should not eat just any and every source of fat found in slaughtered animals. Certain fats like suet are to be given away, especially given over to God. Perhaps this could mean that some fats are so dangerous that no human, even those not belonging to our particular religious communities, should consume them; only God can stomach them—not that God eats, of course. On the other hand, many religious traditions teach that we need not avoid all animal fats, if we choose to eat animals or their products in the first place. The theological challenge, then, is to eat only those fats that are theologically and biologically good for us; anything more would be imprudent and even impudent.

## SALT

The third ingredient we crave perhaps to our detriment is salt. According to the contemporary molecular gastronomist Hervé This, salt plays a critical role in making things taste and smell. Adding salt to soup increases its ionic strength, freeing odorous molecules and thereby enhancing its flavor. Similarly, sodium ions suppress bitterness, making otherwise unpalatable foods edible.[43] Such science corroborates the prophet Job's observation that tasteless food cannot be eaten without salt.[44] According to a *hadith* teaching attributed to Mohammad, salt is the best seasoning.[45]

Salt makes a meal culinarily worthy of consumption but also imbues food with political and theological substance. For example, sharing salt is a way to ensure loyalty between a sovereign and the people, much as God promises an enduring "covenant of salt" to the Levitical caste.[46] In modern terms, salt seals deals.

Jesus, as recorded in the Synoptic Gospels—Matthew, Mark, and Luke—concurs with Job: salt is good when tasted. But salt is more than just a physical, soluble crystal; it is a symbol, and a subversively powerful one at that. Salt's symbolism merits some attention here.[47]

Jesus calls his followers "salt of the earth,"[48] granules as biologically underfoot as they were sociopolitically: they were the meek, the impoverished, the hungry, the persecuted. Jesus hereby brilliantly transforms salt's associations. Whereas in the Hebrew Bible terrestrial salt is connected with desolation and despondency and thus theologically flavored negatively, for Jesus its earthy, or humus, nature reflects the theopolitical humility he champions.[49] In a way, Jesus inverts salt's divine ionic valence.

But what if the people Jesus so loves lose their saltiness? Haughty and no longer humble, can they be redeemed? Jesus's mind is split on this point. Luke says Jesus teaches that when salt has lost its saltiness, it is fit neither for the soil nor for fertilizer; it is trash.[50] In Matthew's account, Jesus is even more severe: tasteless salt is no good whatsoever and should be thrown out and trampled underfoot.[51] It would seem that saltless—that is, tasteless—people cannot and should not be redeemed.

Yet through Mark, Jesus insists, "For everyone will be salted with fire. Salt is good, but if salt has lost its saltiness, how can you season it? Have salt in yourselves, and be at peace with one another."[52] In the ultimate fiery judgment, all people will be salted, just as all sacrifices were salted when put atop the flaming altar in the Temple in Jerusalem.[53] Until that ethereal end time, however, Jesus instructs everyone to be salty, to be earthy collaborators, as if in a social covenant of salt. If you *are* not salty—that is, if you *are* not humble—by nature or by sociohistorical circumstance, then you should act *as if* you were. For it is humility and not haughtiness that preserves peaceful relations. Salt, he well knew, is a preservative. (It even preserves itself: salt can be evaporated back into its crystalline form after being dissolved.) Sugar, by contrast, often leads to fermentation, and fat brings on rancidity. If the relationship between the people and God is to endure the vagaries of time and space, it will need all the persevering properties possible.

However meaningful this spiritual prescription may be, it lacks precision. It remains vague on how much humility—or salt—is healthy in any regard: spiritually, biologically, socially. Sure, salt enhances a food's taste and can ensure rightful relations among humankind and the gods. The ancient Greeks knew this before Jesus, and Mohammad taught this afterward.[54] The quantitative question remains: How much salt suffices to activate the necessary ingredients, be they biological (such as yeast in dough) or spiritual (as in humility)? Too little salt will be ineffective for these physical and metaphysical purposes. The Talmudic rabbis similarly worried insufficient salt would fail to extract all the blood from a piece of meat, risking quick spoilage and contravening the biblical insistence that all animal blood is God's.[55]

Just as too little salt and humility risks physical, social, and religious dangers, too much salt is similarly hazardous. The individual person would risk hypertension, among other ailments. Environmentally, too much salt compromises a land's capacity to produce. Supersaturated liquids produce silt (itself a word derived from *salt*), a problematic sediment for soups and rivers alike. Sprinkling too much salt upon a meal not only spoils its palatability but is a gesture of impoliteness.[56] As Joshua Ben Sirah taught in the second century BCE, "From the beginning, good things were created for the good, but for sinners good things and bad. The basic necessities of human life are water and fire and iron and salt and wheat flour and milk and honey, the blood of the grape and oil and clothing. All these are good for the godly, but for sinners they turn into evils."[57] For those predisposed to waywardness, salt may be more than evil: it can damn.

Not all is lost, however. Salt can also save. Salt can detoxify deadly waters, just as it cleanses newborns.[58] The Talmudic rabbis observed, "The world can live without wine, but the world cannot live without water. The world can live without pepper, but the world cannot live without salt."[59] A similar teaching is found in the Islamic textual tradition: "And to 'Aishah's question, 'O Messenger of Allah, what are the things which are not permissible to withhold?' Mohammad replied: 'Water, salt and fire.' She said: 'O Messenger of Allah, we know what water is, but what about salt and fire?' He said: 'O Humaira', whoever gives fire (to another), it is as if he has given in charity all the food that is cooked on that fire. And whoever gives salt, it is as if he has given in charity all that the salt makes good.'"[60] Salt makes the necessary (consumable foods) good: it makes food taste, literally; and it makes food theologically desirable, or tasteful.

Salt improves not just meals but relations. Philo of Alexandria, a first-century CE Hellenistic Jewish philosopher, insisted that when the biblical Joseph received his brothers in Egypt, he gave them a meal of bread and salt, by then an old sign of friendship.[61] Giving salt is a gesture of hospitality.

Given all these powerful properties of salt, it is unsurprising that Rav, a third-century CE rabbi, simply declares, "A meal without salt is not a meal."[62]

As with sweets and fats, salt is more than a mere tasty item. It has symbolic theological features and social capacities. It can damn and damage just as it can save a soul and salve a wound. Have some salt, but to avoid undesirable consequences refrain from oversalting. Curiously and consistently across these traditions, sharing salt establishes an unbreakable bond, be it a vertical relationship between people and God or between a populace and a human sovereign, or a horizontal relation between compatriots or hosts and guests. Whether it is for physiological, social, or theological goals, giving some salt away to others is laudable. Indeed, sacrificing one's salt intake is the tasteful thing to do.

# 11

## SHARING

*Rabbi Ila'i said, "By three things is a person known:*
*by his cup [koso], by his purse [kiso],*
*and by his anger [ka'aso]."*

—Babylonian Talmud, *'Eruvin* 65b (fifth to seventh century CE)

T his ancient rabbinic maxim observes that three activities profoundly influence our reputations. One is how we handle our emotional lives. Short-tempered or long-suffering, our emotions impact
how others view and treat us. Another is how we manage our finances,
such as whether we are extravagant, stingy, or generous. For better and
for worse, because knowing what someone earns is rare but witnessing
someone's spending habits is easy, others take note of our expenditures.
Perhaps most surprising, the third way we impact our reputation is how
we drink and eat. Our personal consumptive habits express a great deal
about our values and virtues, that is, our taste.

Our eating, no less than our emotions and economics, demonstrates
our ethics. Insofar as eating is profoundly personal and inwardly oriented, as this book argues, it is also at the same time undeniably collective
and outwardly significant. Appreciating how eating is also a collective enterprise is best begun from the inside. Along the way we will uncover
several paradoxes of eating.

Though the alimentary canal has long been studied around the world,
our overall understanding of how it works remains in nascent stages.
Knowing that microorganisms exist most everywhere and even in our
bodies is relatively recent in science, primarily because they are exceed-
ingly small. Since they cannot be seen by the unaided human eye, they
are called subocular. Most civilizations in antiquity did not think they
existed; for them, only the visible world and the more than visible world
(the realms of the deities) were of most concern.

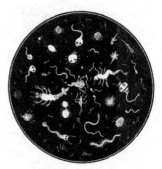

**FIGURE 11.1**

"*Animalculae* in Water," 1846, *Scientific American* 2, no. 3 (October 10): 22.

Yet the subocular could be imagined even if it could not be directly seen. Ultra-small entities were first hypothesized by the Roman scholar Marcus Terentius Varro in 30 BCE. In a three-volume treatise on agricultural issues, Varro advised building a farmhouse facing away from a river: "Note also if there be any swampy ground . . . because certain minute animals (*animalculae*), invisible to the eye, breed there, and, borne by the air, reach the inside of the body by way of the mouth and nose, and cause diseases which are difficult to be rid of."[1] Already, it seems, a connection had been made between these tiny living things and human health, but it would take another millennium and a half before these puny animals were discovered by a man who, of all things, sold drapes.

To see the thread of his cloths better, the Dutchman Antonie Philips van Leeuwenhoek (1632–1723) melted glass into spheres and used those bent lenses to refract what previously had been invisible into the realm of the visible. Bending and grinding glass to see the invisible, whether far off or nearby, was a popular activity in early seventeenth-century Netherlands. Zacharias Jansen, Galileo Galilei, Cornelius Drebbel, Baruch Spinoza, Christiaan Huygens, and others were tinkerers, thinkers, and scientists who helped develop the *vitreus oculum* (glass eye), or what would come to be known as the microscope.[2] Van Leeuwenhoek's devoted attention to the incredibly small enabled him to discover (among many other things) single-celled organisms that he called *animalcules*.

Curious about where such tiny creatures might exist, Leeuwenhoek looked deeply at material taken from his own mouth and from his feces. Upon discovering myriad microorganisms in these materials, he posited that they exist even deeper inside humans. The idea of the human microbiome was thus born.[3]

Gaining access to and studying our internal microbiota, especially those in the gut, proved challenging. Only in recent decades has technology improved enough to identify the existence, diversity, and quantity of the human microbiome. Thanks to the Human Genome Project, scientists have been able to study the genome of this internal microbiota world.

Estimates range wildly about how many microorganisms exist inside us. There could be as few as 10 trillion or as many as 100 trillion symbiotic microbial cells in each person.[4] While some guess that microbial cells outnumber human cells in our body 10:1, recent studies suggest the ratio is more balanced, perhaps even as close as 4:3.[5] Regardless, the vast majority of these foreign cells exist in our guts.

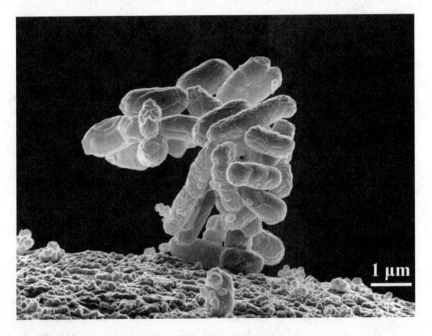

**FIGURE 11.2**

*Escherichia coli* bacteria, magnified here 10,000 times, is a regular member of the human gut microbiome; only a few strains of E. coli cause food poisoning. U.S. Department of Agriculture, Agricultural Research Service, *Wikimedia Commons*, March 2005, https://commons.wikimedia.org/wiki/File:E_coli_at_10000x,_original.jpg.

Appreciation of the importance of gut microorganisms is still in its infancy. Consider just the genetic material this will involve. While humans have about 22,000 genes, the human gut microbiome may have as many as 3.3 million nonredundant genes.[6] Understanding how all these genes work per microorganism remains an unfinished task. Knowing with much clarity how and why they interact with the human organism in which they reside promises to be an ongoing project for a long while.

Yet we do know some things about our relationships with our gut guests. We now know, for example, that gut flora have both commensal and mutualistic relations with us. They simultaneously benefit us and derive benefit from us. Some help ferment chyle, the foodstuff released by the stomach into the intestines, while others synthesize vitamins, metabolize bile, and protect the gut from injury.

Even though our knowledge is far from comprehensive, we can say without exaggeration that the importance of gut microorganisms to human digestion cannot be overstated. These tiny organisms influence human metabolism, human morphology, and even the human psyche. They have a profound impact on obesity.[7] They also affect such psychiatric issues as anxiety, depression, autism-spectrum disorder, obsessive-compulsive disorder, and memory abilities.[8] Yet the relationship is not always a one-way street, from the microbes to us. Evidence is now accruing that the human brain communicates back to these microbiota in ways that, while still mysterious, regulate bodily health.[9]

Such recent evidence speaks to an age-old relationship. We humans, no less than our antecedent species, coevolved with these microorganisms. We need them to survive and thrive, just as they need us for the same. Their help from within enables us to eat the world-not-us in the ways we do. They enable *Homo sapiens* to be metabolically plastic, that is, extremely adaptable to a diverse range of diets.[10] Some of us eat predominantly blubber and animal proteins, whereas others rely exclusively on fruits and vegetables and little else. That the human body can adapt to these dramatically different diets and still thrive is due, in part, to the little helpers in our guts.

While we may be individual ingesters of the world around us, we are not and never have been autonomous digesters. Digestion is and always has been a collaborative effort, from the outside (fellow foragers, hunters, farmers, cooks, etc.) to the inside. We are co-metabolizers. However frequently we may think so, we never dine alone.

Hence the next paradox of eating: eating involves being host and guest at the same time. This inextricable link is forged in the very words themselves. Etymologically, in old French the word *hoste* meant "guest, stranger, and foreigner" as well as "host." Further back, *hospes* in Latin combined *hostis*, meaning "stranger" and *pasco*, "to feed." Thus we get *hospitality, hospitable*, and *hostel*, ways to welcome strangers, as well as *hostile* and *hostility*, ways to push others away. This interrelationship is evident in Hebrew, too. A guest is *'oreaḥ*; a host is *m'areaḥ*, and a meal is *'aruḥa*; all these words share the same three-letter root (*aleph, reish, ḥet*) from the verb meaning "to travel, journey, wander."

These three languages conjoin these experiences and relations. Being a guest who eats, being a host who feeds, being food that is eaten are all interrelated phenomena. Indeed, these words inspire the contemporary scholar of renaissance food David Goldstein to wonder, "Do you feed the guest, or does the guest feed on you?"[11] Or as Leon Kass puts it, "What is the proper treatment of the stranger? In the extreme case, shall you feed him or eat him?"[12] My eating, as guest or host, implicates you, or, says Kass, my eating informs and incorporates you just as it does me. It thus behooves all of us to pay attention to these relations as they can enable us to eat well, live, or not.

Eating is thus never a solipsistic endeavor that involves only me. My eating impacts a whole host (pun intended) of other creatures: those within no less than those nearby and far off. Just as we share our alimentary canals with so many others, we also share the external side of eating with many others. Whereas those internal others are unsightly and invisible, these external ones are not. Figuring out how to interact with them even as we eat is one of life's greatest challenges. As Rabbi Ilai' says, considering anger and emotions in general is integral to living well. So too is the way one organizes and regulates one's wallet and table. Sharing one's vital food bespeaks one's values and virtues. It is a gesture of hospitality and thus necessarily an ethical enterprise.

## BREAKING BREAD I

Many examples can be found in religious traditions to demonstrate the innate interconnections between hosting others and feeding them. Think, for example, of Abraham and Sarah bustling about to make a meal for the three angelic wanderers (Genesis 18). Or of Joseph giving food to the very brothers who sold him into slavery those many years earlier (Genesis 42). In the medieval period, of the four chapters Al-Ghazālī writes on eating, three of them pertain to the rules of eating with others and of hospitality.[13] And Rabbi Bahya devotes a chapter to similar topics in his treatise on eating.

Perhaps the most famous religious depiction of hospitality is Jesus's last meal, in which he instructs his disciples to set up the Passover seder in someone else's house. When they do, the roles get mixed up: the householder host is absent, the guests prepare the banquet, and through his own teachings Jesus becomes the very food everyone is to consume.[14] Jesus even remarks on the difficulty of figuring out which role is more important: "For who is greater, the one who reclines (at the table) or the one who serves? Is it not the one reclining (at the table)? But I am among you as one who serves."[15]

When Jesus breaks the bread, blesses it, and instructs his beloved disciples that it is no longer bread but his own essence and all there should consume it, he insists that the stuff of his life and the stuff of the bread he holds are indistinguishable; their essential substance has been changed. Such transubstantiation enables him to be the consummate host, literally and figuratively: he is that host that is to be consumed by all his guests, and not just this time but anytime and anywhere.

Many centuries passed before this idea of Jesus being consumable took root in Christian communities. Caroline Walker Bynum, a contemporary American scholar of history, avers that the cult of the sacrament or eucharistic host began only in the twelfth century CE. Then Juliana of Cornillon, a canoness in the Premonstratensians, or Norbertine order, worked for decades to solidify its stature, and with the help of Pope Urban IV established in 1264 the feast of Corpus Christi on the Thursday following Pentecost. A motivating theology behind this devel-

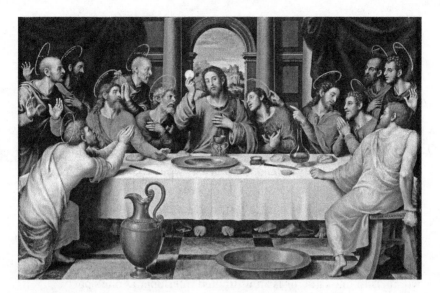

**FIGURE 11.3**

Juan de Juanes, *Last Supper*, 1562.

opment was the idea that "to eat God . . . was finally to become suffering flesh with his suffering flesh; it was to imitate the cross."[16] This desire to be like and with Jesus even unto the end remains compelling.
Hence seeing the host ascend to the church altar, watching it be raised
and praised by priests, and eating it became central components of
proper Catholic worship.

Breaking and sharing bread is hereby elevated as the essential gestures
of hospitality. Sharing bread becomes so enmeshed with hospitality that,
at least for the early rabbis, it may be demanded from any host, even from
royalty themselves. Consider this rabbinic comment upon Hannah's passionate prayer for a child: "By what parable may Hannah's petition be il-
lustrated? By the one of a king of flesh and blood who made a feast for his
servants. A poor man came and, standing by the doorway, begged them,
'Give me a morsel of bread,' but no one heeded him. So he forced his way
into the presence of the king and said, 'My lord king, out of the entire
feast you have made, is it so difficult in your sight to give me one morsel
of bread?'"[17] The chutzpah of this beggar is undeniable. Still, his frustration with the scenario is instructive. His demand was not about justice,

though. He had no right to the food being served at that feast since he was not an invited guest. Because he did not desire to be in that company, his was not a demand for equality. Rather, the beggar's assertion was a moral one. He was more concerned about equity, about securing a reasonable or fair share of food (he just wanted one morsel!) to sustain himself until his next meal. His need to eat was no less and no greater than any other's at that festive occasion; all he sought was enough nutriment to suffice him for now. Surely the feast exceeded everyone's needs, so providing that one morsel would be easy. Indeed, that morsel would be morally expected.

This midrash, commenting on Hannah's prayer for a child, thus binds together the themes of host, guest, and food as well as hospitality and maternity, even of gestation itself. As discussed in chapter 3 regarding the eater, Levinas connects gestation and hospitality. To be hospitable is to feed another, to meet the other's needs, whether that other is in one's womb, is in one's gut, or is an uninvited interloper at one's party.

## BREAKING BREAD II

Central to the above hospitality stories is bread:

- Abraham says to his guests, "And let me fetch a morsel of *bread* that you may refresh yourselves."[18]
- Joseph had a feast of *bread* prepared for his brothers, just as he had before they sold him into slavery.[19]
- Jesus identifies with the *bread* in his hands.

Bread also features in exchanges between Jacob and Esau, Rebecca and Jacob, and innumerably between God and the Israelite people.[20]

Why bread? Of all the foodstuffs we could eat, why is bread so critical to hospitality? Perhaps because, as we read in the second creation story, God insists that it is *for bread* that humans will thereafter sweat.[21] Already from the get-go, bread is identified as that foodstuff that demarcates humankind as an eater unlike any other creature. It is, in a way, a marker of what it means to be human. No other creature, as far as I know, bakes bread. (Some animals might make dough by combining ingredients into paste-like concoctions, but these are hardly what we could reasonably call proto-breadlike recipes.) Might we find bread so alluring because it requires a kind of fermentation, not unlike the fermented drinks that purified liquids? Or maybe it is because baking sparks the Maillard reaction that forms a crust of enticing odors and tastants, thereby signaling that the bread is ready for consumption.

Another plausible reason for bread's centrality to these and so many other classic stories about eating is that it can be easily shared. Bread is what I can rip, break, bring into myself, and yet share with another. Indeed, I should.

To appreciate this, consider that Jews read Isaiah chapter 58 on Yom Kippur, the holiest day in the Jewish calendar, during which they fast for at least twenty-five hours to repent for their waywardness and insensitivity to the plight of others. Levinas comments on this passage by speaking about "the immediacy of the sensible," by which he means that the way you and I experience the world, the ways in which we sense it all, is incredibly proximal: our sensed world is very close to us, bodily speaking. What he finds is that even as we sense the world and enjoy our experiences sensing it, we are also simultaneously frustrated by it. The sensible world is not always enjoyable, nor can it all be enjoyed simultaneously.

Though this frustration perplexes Levinas, it informs a central piece of his overall argument that ethics precedes all else:

> The immediacy of the sensible is the immediacy of enjoyment and its frustration. It is the gift painfully torn up, and in the tearing up, immediately spoiling this very enjoyment. It is not a gift of the heart, but of the bread from one's mouth, of one's own mouthful of bread. It is the openness, not only of one's pocketbook, but of the doors of one's home, a "sharing of your bread with the famished," a "welcoming of the wretched into your house" (Isaiah 58). The immediacy of the sensibility is the for-the-other of one's own materiality; it is the immediacy or the proximity of the other.[22]

The immediacy of the world that we sense necessarily includes the person whose hunger we cannot ignore. This other is so close that we can and should reach out, though not with an empty hand. Our hand should include the bread we have just ripped from our own mouths. It turns out that this gesture constitutes one's own identity. By "giving to the other of the bread out of one's own mouth . . . the identity of the subject is here brought out, not by a rest on itself, but by a restlessness that drives me outside of the nucleus of my substantiality."[23] By wresting this crust of bread from my own mouth and giving it to another I ensure that my identity has meaning beyond myself. I become me by giving away some of my own food.

Though he meditated at length upon it, Levinas did not originate the idea of ripping a morsel of bread from one's mouth to nourish someone else. This gesture can be seen in a tenth-century midrash on the biblical phrase that God gave Moses two tablets of the pact atop Mt. Sinai:

> Thus it is written, *For Adonai gives wisdom, out of* [*God's*] *mouth comes knowledge and discernment* (Proverbs 2:6). Wisdom is great, but greater still is knowledge and discernment. Hence, *For Adonai gives wisdom*; but to him whom God loves, [directly] *out of* [*God's own*] *mouth comes knowledge and discernment.* . . . Rabbi Isaac and Rabbi Levi [interpret this verse]. One said that it can be compared to a rich man's son, who, on returning from school, found a dish of food in front of his father. When the father offered him a piece, the son said: "I would rather have some of that which you yourself are now eating." The father complied, on account of his great love for him, giving him from his own mouth. This illustrates *For Adonai gives wisdom*; but of him whom God loves even more, we read: *Out of* [*God's*] *mouth comes knowledge and discernment.*[24]

Giving wisdom, this midrash suggests, is rather commonplace. Most anyone can share with others illuminating insights and guidance, such as what one should do in particular circumstances. Extending knowledge and discernment is different: these are ways of thinking, analyzing, and problem solving. Giving others these kinds of tools nourishes their cognitive capacities in ways that pithy wisdom does not. For these rabbis, sharing with others such intellectual skills is the same as giving to others the very bread that one is just about to ingest.

This kind of sharing is profoundly intimate. It connects us to others in unique ways that no other relationship can truly imitate. Giving another the bread one consumes expresses deep and great love: it embodies the transmission of life-sustaining thoughts as much as it puts into another's body the nourishment one could have otherwise selfishly hoarded. Consuming less than one can is perhaps the holiest way to think and eat. Whether bread or discernment, by giving it away, *by sharing, one accrues meaning.*

## NEEDING HUNGER

Sharing gives us meaning. The very opportunity to share, though, is contingent upon the existence of others who need or are hungry. Let us consider this complex relationship.

Recall my earlier discussions about appetite, need, and desire. Levinas, like his philosophical predecessors, also differentiates need from desire. On his account, need is a natural mode of existence, a dependence happy because it can be satisfied, just as a void can become filled. A needy body is at the same time dependent upon and liberated from the world. It is dependent upon the external world for its nourishment. Yet that very extraction from the world beyond demonstrates the body's liberation or separation from that external world, since the body drags what is outside inside, into an interior otherwise inaccessible to all else out there. Nourishment, Levinas observes, "as a means of invigoration, is the transmutation of the other into the same, which is the essence of enjoyment; an energy that is other, recognized as other, recognized . . . as sustaining the very act [that is, metabolism] that is directed upon it, become, in enjoyment, my own energy, my strength, me. All enjoyment is in this sense alimentation."[25] Eating en-joys me; it makes me happy. For as I eat, the eaten becomes in part my own energy. Eating enlivens me. Were I a creature with no need to eat, I would know neither enjoyment nor happiness. I would be "a castrated soul," extirpated of need.[26] Whereas Plato understood need to be a simple lack, and Kant viewed it as a kind of passivity, Levinas insists that my need (to eat) constitutes my very happiness: "The human being thrives on his needs; he is happy for his needs."[27]

So here is another paradox of eating: I am happy for my hunger. This is because I *can* satisfy my need for shelter, clothing, food, and water. Most needs are needs of material, and as such, they are within each person's power, at least theoretically. Thus Levinas says, "In need I can sink my teeth into the real and satisfy myself in assimilating the other."[28] This consumption of the materially real makes me happy. In becoming happy, I *am*. Reflecting on Levinas's insights, Goldstein aptly observes that this is "a direct attack on the sentence in which the philosophy of existence might be said to originate, the *cogito ergo sum*."[29] When Levinas claims, "For the I to be means neither to oppose nor to represent something to itself, nor to use something, nor to aspire to something, but to enjoy something," Goldstein summarizes this to mean, "I is not I until I am enjoying. I eat, therefore I am."[30]

Eating demonstrates my individuality and separation from the external world as much as it does my dependence upon and need for that material otherness, and eating makes me happy by incorporating (literally) that paradox. Satisfying my hunger makes me happy.

Of course, I can become so wrapped up in satisfying my hunger, in my own enjoyment, that my whole being, my sense of self, becomes all-consuming. I can become a totality coiled into myself, while the world at large disappears. When I eat, I am happy—and that is all that (increasingly) matters. Moses rails against such haughty consumption: we should never become so full of ourselves.

But is this all? Is eating truly only a hedonistic, self-serving activity satisfying one's incessant need? Could it not be that sating one's hunger makes one both happy and sad?

Consider that the Old English word *sad*, based on the Latin *satis*, means "enough" or "sated." Perhaps alimentary satisfaction can be both enjoyable and saddening simultaneously. Even as eating en-joys me, it encumbers me, burdening me with the materiality of existence and the weighty awareness of this very fact.[31] Hence, another paradox: when eating, we become happy and sad simultaneously.

Whereas my hunger is my need for an other like bread and it can be met by taking that bread into myself, desire is something else entirely. According to Levinas, if need strives for incorporating the physical, desire reaches for the metaphysical: "The other metaphysically desired is not 'other' like the bread I eat, the land in which I dwell, the landscape I contemplate. . . . I can 'feed' on these realities and to a very great extent satisfy myself, as though I had simply been lacking them. Their *alterity* [otherness] is thereby reabsorbed into my own identity as a thinker or a possessor. The metaphysical desire tends toward *something else entirely*, toward the *absolutely other*."[32] Goldstein calls this last sentence a philosophical "slap in the face, positing a sharp discontinuity between the desire for food (which circles back to the self) and 'metaphysical desire,' which breaks out beyond the self toward otherness."[33] In meeting the need for nourishment, eating "coils" the self upon itself: I become sated by incorporating graspable, munchable others, the world-not-me.[34] Why *coil*? It comes from the Latin *colligere*, meaning "to gather together." Eating gathers the world into me, solidifying my material existence.

Metaphysical desire does not coil the self together. It interrupts this reinforcement of the self, breaking the self's boundaries by stretching out to that which can never be assimilated, consumed, or absorbed. Metaphysical desire is always beyond reach: "There is no sinking one's teeth into being, no satiety, but an unchartered future before me."[35] Metaphysical desire opens the self to its own future. Out there in that unknown and unknowable future one's very meaning and identity are available to shape and experience. Our metaphysical desires unfold our identities, whereas our physical needs fold us back into ourselves and can crush us, even sadden us profoundly, if we are not careful.

Return for a moment to Levinas's claim "I can 'feed' on these realities and to a very great extent satisfy myself, as though I had simply been lacking them." The phrase *to a very great extent* is vital. Were material satisfaction achieved completely, it would be an eternal state. It would be unlivable. Stones, for example, have all their needs met. Being always or completely sated would be deadly. Since perfect satisfaction kills, eating the world must satisfy hunger only *to a very great extent*.

A further paradox: Life needs need. In every moment, we need need. Our biological satisfaction must always be incomplete so that we may endure in and through time. "To be sure," Levinas insists, "need is also a dependence with regard to the other, but it is a dependence across time."[36] Need needs time "to convert this *other* into *the same* by labor [by, say, digestion]. . . . For a body that labors everything is not already accomplished, already done; thus to be a body is to have time in the midst of the facts, to be *me* though living in the *other*."[37] Put differently: for a body that digests, everything is not already accomplished, since digestion is the on-going act of extracting energy from without and waste from within. To be a body means requiring time to sort this all out, to incorporate me as distinct from all that other material.

Since I cannot endure for long without satisfying my thirst or my hunger to some degree, I am dependent *through time* on the stuff out there in the world. But *in time*, in this particular moment, in this very instant, I am independent of that stuff. In Kass's words, "The organism is, always, coincident with its materials at any moment, but it is independent of—not tied to—any one collection of stuff over time. Indeed, if organic form ever coincided for any length of time with the exact same collection of molecules, it would have ceased to live. The organism would have become a thing, with exactly the same form-material identity as seen in such inanimate bodies as rocks and crystals."[38] When Levinas puts it this way, "in need I can sink my teeth into the real and satisfy myself in assimilating the other,"[39] he promotes the practice of eating to satisfy one's hunger and not going beyond that.

This hints at yet another paradox: eating well satisfies a need imperfectly. Thus, even as I sink my teeth into this crust of bread, even as I now labor through digestion to satisfy my hunger, *I can never and ought never fully sate my hunger*. This would kill me—physiologically no less than philosophically.

I can live and live best from moment to moment by eating some but not to the fullest extent I can. By eating in this "just right" range, I am able to feed someone else with the food I am not consuming—and this gives my life meaning. "To give, to-be-for another, despite oneself, but in interrupting the for-oneself, is to take the bread out of one's own mouth, to nourish the hunger of another with one's own fasting."[40] My eating, indeed my very being, is meaningful when it presumes your eating, satisfaction, and enjoyment as well: "This sensibility has meaning only as a 'taking care of the other's need,' of his misfortunes and his faults, that is, as a giving. But giving has meaning only as a tearing from oneself despite oneself, and not only *without* me. And to be torn from oneself despite oneself has meaning only as a being torn from the complacency in oneself characteristic of enjoyment, snatching the bread from one's mouth. *Only a subject that eats can be for-the-other.*"[41] Eating thus is a sharing activity. By sharing food, even the food one is about to ingest, one becomes more than an animate creature: one becomes a moral subject. As Brillat-Savarin says, "Digestion is of all the bodily operations the one which has the greatest influence on the moral state of the individual."[42] Through eating we become our moral selves.

That said, feeding others may not be intuitive to every eater. Feeding others comes naturally—to nature. The generosity of the natural world is indisputable. It provides copious foodstuffs for humans and all other species without even so much as a grumble against our ingratitude. We are beneficiaries of nature's largesse not because of our merit but because nature naturally hosts. As the ultimate host, nature feeds its denizen guests before it consumes those very creatures themselves when they finally die. As far as we can tell, nature does not wrestle with whether or how to host. It just does.

Hospitality among humans, however, must be deliberate. It is also an opportunity to demonstrate our very humanity. The other person's hunger, Kass notes, "provides the occasion for our own nobility, for rising above necessity. Feeding oneself is obligatory, but feeding *another* feeder is liberal, that is, free. Necessity is thus the mother also of virtue."[43] Again the maternal tropes of hospitality and gestation, eating and feeding, necessity and ethics, intertwine.

## COMMENSALITY

Manifesting such generosity requires looking across the table. When we sit at the same table with other eaters, we are commensals: *com* is "with" in Latin; *mensa* is "table." Commensality is the act of eating at the same table.

Shared meals are not all alike, of course. We have dinner parties, potlucks, brunches, buffets, barbecues. We have dates over meals, meetings with drinks, water-cooler snack breaks, picnics in the park. Even one eating event has within it several types of meals. Consider the nineteenth-century painting of a children's party by the German Ludwig Knaus. Two cacophonous tables of children dominate the scene. At the smaller one young children are fed by someone older, feed themselves, quarrel over a plate of food, watch another being fed, or feed a nearby cat. A palpable

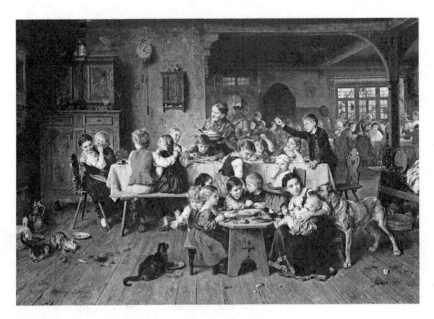

**FIGURE 11.4**

Ludwig Knaus, *Ein Kinderfest* (The Children's Party), 1868.

tension erupts at the larger table as the young man at the right gestures at the other end, where a boy is attempting to steal a kiss from what I presume to be the young man's sister. Of the two who are in the midst of eating, only one uses a utensil. More civilized dining occurs at the distant third table, where adults calmly sup, drink, chat, and are entertained with music. This lively painting depicts an unmistakably clear message: (celebratory) eating is a dynamic, social occasion.

Shared eating is also a site of contestation. Contemporary scholar of food studies and sustainability Alice Julier finds that shared meals "are tied up in particular understandings of difference and inequality, understandings that emerge from the historical and contemporary configuration of gender, race, and class."[44] In every age and in every place we use meals both to distinguish ourselves from others and to provide ourselves with "different skills and relationships that are often specifically useful for their communities." We continuously define and refine ourselves in and by sharing our tables.

This strategy is old. In his study of Renaissance society, Goldstein contends that "eating, commensality, and community were bound together."[45] Medieval Jewish mystics also noted that sharing a festal table necessarily linked tablemates into an identifiable social group.[46] Sharing tables was not always a good idea, however. An ancient warning taught, "When you sit down to dine with a ruler, consider well who is before you. Thrust a knife into your gullet if you have a large appetite. Do not crave for his dainties, for they are counterfeit food."[47] This adage teaches us to pay close attention to the food we eat, how we eat, as well as those with whom we eat. In brief: the eaten, eating, and fellow eaters, all merit our careful attention.

Even while tables are not infinitely expandable and not everyone is welcome at them simply because, in large measure, all cannot physically fit around them, old and enduring notions show that sharing tables is nonetheless important. For example, according to the Benedictine order, the Superior was to make guests comfortable when they arrive and even break his own fast so that the guest not dine alone.[48] Talmudic rabbis tell of an incident of laborers who regularly pooled their bread into a basket and then ate together from that collective bounty. One day an individual had nothing to contribute to that common pot and felt ashamed; the fellow collecting the food that day recognized the situation and pretended to take bread from him so as to protect him from further shame.[49] The rabbinic midrash of King David eating with commoners from a collective pot suggests that the idea of mixing classes over meals may have biblical roots.[50] Sharing meals can transcend class, social norms, and emotions, just as it can cross religious and royal thresholds.

Because commensality or eating at the same table is transformative, Brillat-Savarin distinguishes the pleasures of eating from the pleasures of the table. On his view, the pleasures of eating include the direct sensations of tasting and ingesting and digesting the world. Humans share these experiences with the larger animate kingdom. However, the pleasures of the table are exclusive to humankind. These pleasures are deliberate: they depend upon careful consideration of where eating occurs, with whom, and the preparation of the foods themselves.[51] Since shared meals are highly cogitated events, they are often judiciously choreographed: every culture has its own etiquette, rules, and norms for how to eat, formalities for engaging in conversation, expectations of dress and decorum, plans for sequencing dishes.

I will leave to Kass, Julier, Martha Stewart, Margaret Visser, and their predecessors Emily Post, Brillat Savarin—even before them, Al-Ghazālī and Bahya ben Asher ibn Halawa—the details surrounding the rules of dining together, or etiquette. Rules, expectations, and anticipation tell us how to behave at the collective table, whether with kin or others. Personal manners (fork held this way, use of knife), delivery of food (buffet, plated, family-style), food display (in pots, crockery, crystal), ambiance (music, lighting, art, decor), conversation topics, seating arrangements, clothing, hors d'oeuvres, aperitifs, desserts, drinks, sequencing, pacing, eye contact, vocal volume, and more, all are part of the commensal picture. Evidence of the importance of shared meals to civilization and the care with which people organize and host them is easily seen on ancient vases depicting Greek feasts, in the ornate decorations accompanying Chinese banquets, and in myriad dishes offered at Indian weddings.

At one level commensality provides stimulating pleasure. As Brillat-Savarin says, "Pleasure is enjoyed in almost all its extent when the following conditions are united: good cheer, good wine, a pleasant company, and time."[52] At another level, Serres holds that commensality can be philosophically stimulating: "The title of every banquet should be: sapience and sagacity. Around the table, only sage tongues."[53]

Whether joining together for a good time or for collaboratively investigating good ideas, sharing meals and their accompanying etiquette nourish civilizations, not just individual bodies. To share a meal means to eat well, and conversely, to eat well means to share meals. Go ahead, enjoy some of the repast in front of you, but refrain so that others may partake as well. Such eating makes each individual at the table flourish as much as it does the society of which they are a part. Sharing makes us all thrive. Let us make that choice.

# CONCLUSION

———

*Who is responsible for the power to exploit,*
*for the privilege to consume?*

—Abraham Joshua Heschel, *God in Search of Man* (1993)


*All the labor of man is for his mouth.*

—Ecclesiastes 6:7

# 12

## GO AHEAD, REFRAIN

*Remove your hand from a meal*
*that pleases you.*

—Babylonian Talmud, *Gittin* 70a

The argument to go ahead, eat and refrain is not new, of course. Civilizations millennia ago often zealously guided, goaded, and restricted people to and from consuming what, in their view, was too much. Many of these rules and regulations became known as sumptuary laws.

Consider, for example, some laws enacted by Marcus Porcius Cato (243–149 BCE), who after military service rose as a senator in ancient Rome. He despised Hellenic culture and its ostentatiousness; he feared it would corrupt and erode Rome's conventionalism. Under his leadership Lex Orchia was passed in 181 BCE to limit the number of guests who could be invited to a feast. Two decades later, Lex Fannia was passed, prescribing the kind and value of foods for feasts: one hundred asses were permitted for such important holidays as Ludi Romani, Ludi Plebeii, and Saturnalia, but only thirty for lesser festivals and ten on all other days of the year.[1]

Along with other rules about how much Romans should spend on meals, the kinds of food they should serve, and the quantities they should provide, these laws no doubt delimited ostentatious expenditure and waste. They were not the only laws articulated in the ancient Mediterranean basin to restrain excess.

Look at the many biblical rules about the number of animals to be sacrificed for various holy days.[2] The texts often stipulate that a single dove is to be brought for sacrifice, but sometimes as much as two oxen. The expense of these sacrifices for the Israelites at that time may have been great. Because of this, the text in many places accommodates those who have fewer resources: the poorer are permitted to bring less expensive gifts like grains and oil. These vegetarian gifts will be just as able as the more expensive ones to fulfill the rites of the required sacrifice.

These rules also capped how much people should spend on these sacrifices. To bring more than what was stipulated would have been boastful, even chutzpadic. These rules were, in their way, a form of sumptuary law.

Sumptuary legislations identify a realm of extraordinary luxury that a particular society finds reprehensible. People *could* spend their resources in those ways, say, killing 205 oxen for a wedding instead of the 200 put into law, or bringing three oxen instead of two for a sacrifice at the Temple. Rather, these rules hold that people *should not* spend their resources in those ways. Such expenditure would be too much.

These laws thus divide expenditure into at least two categories. At the upper extreme are those that are deemed excessive, lying beyond what could be supported on social, political, economic, environmental, or theological grounds. They ought to be eschewed, even though some in a particular society could nonetheless afford them. Conspicuous consumption is deemed suspicious consumption. Below that realm are defensible expenditures that society endorses. It is their breach that society enforces.

Sumptuary laws were not neutral, of course. They prevented aristocrats from ostentatious splurging, and they also kept others from spending as if they were aristocrats. Social divisions and class and political privileges were regulated and reinforced through such laws, because the ruling classes, such as the nobility and clergy, often exempted themselves from these very laws. While *they* could spend as extravagantly as they wished, *others* must hold themselves in check. To make things worse, those subject to the rules were often denigrated in part because they were not the rule makers. This meant their ways of living—including their ways of procuring, preparing, and consuming food—were also denigrated. In brief, sumptuary laws, like shared meals, were yet another way for societies to reinforce their stratifications.

Such exemption and discrimination do not apply, however, to the proposal of restraint put forward by this book. Sumptuary laws are helpful to consider for this project insofar as they indicate a long-standing and nearly universal societal impetus to identify and to value (negatively) the realm of the excessive. Extravagance for its own sake is deemed repugnant and ought to be avoided.

We may enjoy luxury at *some* times or in *some* ways. Indeed, many civilizations and cultures identify certain times, places, and reasons for extravagance: holy days, lifecycle events, accomplishments.[3] Those are to be exceptional occasions, however. The rest of the time we should restrain ourselves from such indulgence. To make the point even sharper: most of the time we ought not overindulge.

This holds true of an individual's consumptive practice. Overindulgence, while occasionally permitted in certain communities, would be a maladaptive eating strategy were it to be practiced regularly. Eat some, but less than what one can.

This is of course easier to say than uphold. I acknowledge the difficulty, especially given the contemporary food environment.

The idea is not unique to me. For example, Michael Pollan organizes his top "food rules" into three major categories: eat food, mostly plants, not too much. He offers in this last category some specific strategies that

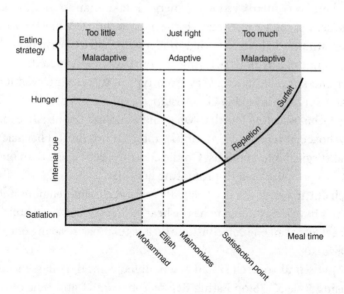

**FIGURE 12.1**

Go ahead, refrain. Envisioning a better diet.

echo the call to eat only until one is satisfied. Rule 54, "Eat Less," is, he admits, "the most unwelcome advice of all." And yet "the scientific case for eating less than you currently do—regardless of whether you are overweight—is compelling. 'Calorie restriction' has repeatedly been shown to slow aging in animals, and many researchers believe it offers the single strongest link between diet and cancer prevention. We eat much more than our bodies need to be healthy, and the excess wreaks havoc—and not just on our weight. When it comes to food, less really is more."[4] Research since the 1930s corroborates this claim in other species.[5] In humans, a recent multisite, randomized clinical trial found that a 25 percent calorie restriction in diet sustained over two years had a substantial positive impact on quality-of-life indices among the moderately overweight.[6] Another conclusion of that study was that no negative effects on health-related quality of life, such as sex life, perceived and real health, sleep, relationships, or overall emotional health, occurred. Other scholars observed that moderate caloric restriction in humans dramatically improves metabolically-related conditions that cause morbidity, disability, and even mortality.[7] Another study concluded that since more people can adhere to regularly reducing energy intake than to dieting that includes fasting, caloric restriction is the most sustainable dietary strategy.[8] Further studies demonstrate that moderately restrictive diets positively impact longevity by both delaying the onset of age-related diseases like cancer and stimulating recovery from typical disease interventions via pills and surgery.[9] In many circumstances, eating less can lead to living longer.[10] That is, eating less than what one could has few negative medical or psychosocial repercussions, unlike many, if not most, pharmacological and surgical interventions. On the contrary, eating less than one's capacity has profound health-promoting qualities.

Such cutting-edge science belatedly reinforces what religions and philosophies have long known to be the heartiest, healthiest, and holiest way to eat: eat less than one can consume on a regular basis, saving one's feasting for feasts.

If you do find yourself seated at a bounteous meal, Pollan encourages exercising Rule 55, "Stop Eating Before You're Full," and Rule 61, "Leave Something on Your Plate." For the latter, *not* cleaning your plate will "help you eat less in the short term and develop self-control in the long."

This suggestion, "Better to go to waste than to waist," orients the eater to external cues. The plate becomes the arbiter of how much one should eat. Why not put less on one's plate in the first place? Why waste anything if it can be avoided?

The other rule, by contrast, orients eaters to their own bodies. Instead of eating until one is full, many cultures and traditions teach people to stop before reaching that point of repletion. In Pollan's words: "To say 'I'm hungry' in French you say '*J'ai faim*'—'I have hunger'—and when you are finished, you do not say that you are full, but '*Je n'ai plus faim*'—'I have no more hunger.' That is a completely different way of thinking about satiety. When we ask our children, 'Are you full?' we're teaching them to eat more than they need to be satisfied. Better to ask, 'Are you satisfied?' The same goes for you: Ask yourself not, Am I full? But, Is my hunger gone? You'll find that moment arrives several bites sooner."[11] This suggestion is perhaps Pollan's most profound since it relies not on external cues but on internal awareness. Anyone who eats can probably entertain the question "Is my hunger gone? Am I satisfied?" And the answer can be as universal as it is individualized. Socioeconomic circumstances need not be a factor in raising and answering this kind of question.

Consider biblical Ruth. An outsider by gender, class, and religion, she nonetheless is invited to a meal by Boaz, the quintessential landowning male insider. "At mealtime, Boaz said to her, 'Come here and partake of the meal, and dip your morsel in the vinegar.' So she sat down beside the [other] reapers. He handed her roasted grain, and she ate her fill and had some left over."[12] Ruth resumed working in the fields and at the day's end returned to Naomi, her mother-in-law, and gave those leftovers to her.[13] If Ruth, of the outcast and disenfranchised poor, can eat according to this strategy of "go ahead, refrain," and thereby ensure that others can also meet their bodily needs, then all the more so can, and perhaps should, those who are more socioeconomically secure.

Turning our individual consumptive attention inward is critical to eating well. Yet we cannot eat well by responding only to internal cues. We must do both: pay attention to our bodies and to the world around us. As Goldstein puts it, "In all cases, eating urges us toward a relational understanding of the self, which in turn forces us to consider the ethical ramifications of our constitution by and in the world."[14]

Eating well in this manner avoids many pitfalls that trouble other interventions that address eating directly or merely its visible and insidious symptoms, like obesity. Prescriptive diets notoriously fail to produce long-term weight loss, and similarly, diets to gain weight often endanger participants because they presume a generic body, not the peculiarities of my or your or any particular body. Pills, another popular strategy, similarly endanger consumers not only with potent, morbid, and even mortal side effects but also because of habituation: few people achieve a weight or eating practice that is sustainable without taking those pills. Autonomy or independent homeostasis remains elusive in such pharmacological programs.

The failures of these nonsurgical interventions are matched by surgical ones. Bariatric surgery in all its forms may drastically reduce a body's weight and reshape its morphology in the short run but hardly impacts a person's eating habits. While certain techniques are new, bariatric surgery is an old strategy. Consider this Talmudic story: A rabbi was given a sleeping potion, brought into a marble chamber, his stomach cut open, and baskets of fat were removed from his gut. The fat was taken out into the sun for several months during the summer, yet it did not putrefy because it was pure fat and had no blood in it.[15] Though it is unclear what happened to that rabbi postsurgery, then as today, any and all invasive surgery incurs risk of infections, ruptures, and more, not to mention heavy monetary costs, time in hospitals and clinics, and emotional turmoil for the patient and those caring for the patient.

Consider, too, this proposal in light of the four central tenets or principles of modern bioethics: autonomy, beneficence, non-maleficence, and justice. Eating just enough or until satisfied relies solely and exclusively on each eater. Each person's autonomy is championed. A new homeostasis is achieved as the body adapts to its new energy-acquisition patterns; it is beneficent to each body. It has no risk of exogenous, sometimes nauseating, debilitating, or lethal side effects; with so few potential harms, its maleficence is negligible. And as it is far cheaper and accessible than most other reactive interventions, this proactive eating strategy is just—for individuals as for society as a whole.[16] Whereas other strategies excel in one principle or another, only this proposal upholds all four.

"Go ahead, eat and refrain" may be an imperfect proposal, however, because, in part, it relies upon each eater to know what it means to eat, how one eats, and why. Many may not want to investigate these issues or know themselves so well. Still, the perfect should not be the enemy of the good. It is a place to start.

Indeed, as Wendell Berry observed, it is perhaps the only place to start. In his view, modern food industrialists "have by now persuaded millions of consumers to prefer food that is already prepared. They will grow, deliver, and cook your food for you and (just like your mother) beg you to eat it. That they do not yet offer to insert it, prechewed, into our mouth is only because they have found no profitable way to do so. We may rest assured that they would be glad to find such a way. The ideal industrial food consumer would be strapped to a table with a tube running from the food factory directly into his or her stomach."[17]

While I do not agree that all people or companies involved with providing food to our modern societies operate with this goal in mind, I do take Berry's point. The modern food environment is fairly hostile to individuals becoming knowledgeable about where their food comes from, much less being in control of their eating. Berry describes this situation as a trap of industrialism in which merchandise is let into our societies and cities, but consciousness is not permitted to come out. "How does one escape this trap? Only voluntarily, the same way that one went in: by restoring one's consciousness of what is involved in eating; by reclaiming responsibility for one's own part in the food economy."[18] Here I agree with Berry. We each must individually and voluntarily liberate our consciousness, especially in regard to eating. This is no manifesto per se, but a call to act for our very lives.

We, the eaters the world, need not unite to resist the insidiousness of the contemporary food environment, though that is not a bad idea. Collective action has always proven powerful. Rather, we, the eaters of the world, need to voluntarily empower ourselves individually with the consciousness of our own eating. We should know ourselves as eaters with peculiar physiological needs, philosophical ideas, and theological desires. What we will find is that eating well is an individual and individualizing endeavor. Eating well is a choice available to us several times daily. How and why we make our consumptive choices reflect and reinforce our identity and values. For all these reasons, how and why we eat are two of the most urgent and pressing ethical questions of our very existence, and their answers lie daily in our own hands and mouths.

# NOTES

## PREFACE

1. Crane 2013.

## 1. FULL OF OURSELVES

1. Brillat-Savarin 1999:45.
2. Ecclesiastes 2:24. Bible translations follow the *New Jewish Publication Society of America Tanakh* (1985).
3. According to the *Oxford English Dictionary*, being full or replete with food and drink has Old English roots in the eleventh-century Paris Psalter. Jonathan Swift (1766:85b) may have been the first to coin the phrase "I am full" in connection with food, in a letter he wrote in 1710. A Google search of published materials for the phrase "I'm full" shows that its prevalence increased dramatically in the mid-twentieth century, just after the phrase "Fill 'er up" came into vogue. https://books.google.com/ngrams /graph?content=%22+Fill+her+up+%22%2C%22+I%E2%80%99m+full+%22&year _start=1900&year_end=2000&corpus=15&smoothing=3&share&.
4. "The pleasure of satisfaction would express the reestablishment of a natural plenitude. And yet this whole psychology of need is a bit hasty. It too quickly interprets the insufficiency of need as an insufficiency of being. Thus it assumes a metaphysics in which need is characterized in advance as an emptiness in a world where the real is identified with the full" (Levinas 2003:58).
5. For more on the philosophy of organic existence, see Jonas 1966, 1984; Schwartz and Wiggins 2010; Scodel 2003.
6. Pavlov 1904.
7. Nietzsche 2001:34.
8. Ibid.

## 2. DEPRIVATION AND GLUTTONY

1. Philippians 3:19. See also Romans 16:18. New Testament translations are from the New Revised Standard Version.
2. Hill 2011:1.
3. Griffith (2004) offers an engaging study of such mind-sets in American Christianity.
4. For but one study, see Ludwig et al. 2011.
5. Miller 1997:93.
6. Murtagh and Ludwig 2011:206.
7. See Leitch and Geliebter (2015) for additional perspectives on these and other influences.
8. Murtagh and Ludwig 2011:206.
9. See Burgand 2009.
10. Leitch and Geliebter 2015:86.
11. See, for example, Smith and Dockray 2006.
12. See, for example, those surveyed in Conason 2015.
13. Shulḥan Aruch, *Orach Chayim* 618.1, 618.15.
14. Sermon 20, Ninth Sermon for the December Fast, pars. 2–3, *Patrologia Latina* 54, cols. 189–90, quoted in Bynum 1987:31. The original Latin can be found here: https://books.google.com/books?id=9fgQAAAAYAAJ&vq=189&pg=PA187#v=onepage&q&f=false.
15. Isaiah 58:3–5.
16. Babylonian Talmud (hereafter BT), *Ta'anit* 11a–b.
17. See the fascinating discussion in Bynum (1987) about how fasting, abstinence, and asceticism were variously conceived and perceived in medieval European cultures and religions.
18. Qur'an 2:183–84, Sahih translation.
19. See Leitch and Geliebter 2015:92–94.
20. Nathan's Famous, "Nathan's Famous International Hot Dog Eating Contest," http://www.nathansfamous.com/hot-dog-eating-contest.
21. Major League Eating, http://www.majorleagueeating.com/index.php. These events are hosted by the International Federation of Competitive Eating (IFOCE). Another significant organization in this field is All Pro Eating (APE). Alka-Seltzer is a frequent corporate sponsor of these events. See also Eats Feats news feed about competitive eating.
22. Aristotle, *Nicomachean Ethics*, III:11.
23. See discussion in Hill 2011:58–59.
24. *St. Benedict's Rule for Monasteries*, Rule 39. See Doyle 1948:58–59.
25. Luke 21:34–36.
26. See Aquinas 1947: part II, Q 148. See also discussion in Thompson 2015:82–83.
27. Kant 1996b:180.
28. Kant 1996b:180–81.
29. Kant 1996b:176.

30. See Douglas 1972, discussed below.
31. Kant 1996b:177.
32. Miller 1997:97.
33. Miller 1997:98.
34. Luke 12:22–23; Matthew 6:25.
35. Luke 12:30–31; Matthew 6:32–33.

## 3. THE EATER

1. *Phaedo* 64d.
2. *Phaedo* 67e.
3. For more on Epicurus, see discussion in Thompson 2015:81ff.
4. Descartes 1637: part 4; 1644: part 1, §7.
5. Bahya ben Asher ibn Halawa in the fourteenth century, for example, is a clear dualist when he says, "The righteous person ought to direct his mind when he is eating only to the fact that the bodily meal by which he will sustain his body for the moment is so that his soul with it may show its powers and realize them in action, and by this prepare the eternal meal by which it will be sustained forever" (*Shulḥan Shel Arba*, Second Gate, p. 11).
6. Spinoza 1994:128.
7. Spinoza 1994:224–25 (IV, P45, S).
8. See discussion in Klein 2003:195.
9. Ecclesiastes 2:25. Biblical quotes come from the New Jewish Publication Society edition of the Tanakh.
10. Ecclesiastes 5:16.
11. Ecclesiastes 5:16–18.
12. Brillat-Savarin 1999:3.
13. Levinas 1998a:75.
14. Levinas 1998a:56.
15. Levinas 1998b:10.
16. Levinas 1998b:11.
17. Levinas 1998a:72. Might he be reflecting on his experience as a prisoner of war in Nazi-occupied France? Such a belligerent context is suggestive.
18. Some might be tempted to add an anthropocentric phrase like "and this sets us apart from the nonhuman world." Increasing evidence from ethology and other fields concerning animals challenge such claims to human exceptionalism. See, for example, Crane 2015. Evidence of plants, trees especially, sharing vital nutrients is also growing. See Wohlleben 2016.
19. Levinas 1998a:74, emphasis added.
20. Levinas 1987:64.
21. Goldstein 2010:36.

## 4. THE EATEN

1. Aristotle agrees that the very concept of food is complicated. See his *De Anima* (The Soul), II.5.
2. Berry 2009.
3. Wirzba 2011:74–75.
4. For a colorful, fact-filled consideration of animal waste, see Foer 2009:174–78.
5. See the many resources at Esselstyn's website, www.engine2diet.com.
6. Wright 1999:xv.
7. Wright 1999: back cover.
8. See, for example, Bynum 1987; Jung 2004; Wirzba 2011; Rosenblum 2010, 2016.
9. Brillat-Savarin 1999:65.
10. Kass 1999:22.
11. Matthew 15:11 (NRSV). Regarding the capacity of what emerges from the mouth to defile, see Matthew 15:18–20. See also Mark 7:14–20. Contrast this with Moses's teaching that "man may live on anything that Adonai decrees"—that is, on anything that comes from God's mouth (Deuteronomy 8:3).
12. John 6:27.
13. John 6:48–51. See also John 6:35; 1 Corinthians 10:16, 11:24. Elsewhere Jesus describes himself as a vine, God the gardener, and the people the fruit of the vine—another metaphoric use of food (John 15:1–4).
14. Moses informs the Israelites that manna would spoil (Exodus 16:19–24).
15. John 6:52–58.
16. See Leviticus 26:21–33; Deuteronomy 28:53–57; Jeremiah 19:9; Lamentations 4:10, 2:20; Ezekiel 5:5–12. See also 2 Kings 6:24–30, discussed below.
17. Interestingly, the Qur'an and classic hadith literature never explicitly identify or outlaw cannibalism. See Qur'an 2:173, 16:115; *Dawud* 27.3798, 27.3808, 27.3780, 27.3781. All translations of the Qur'an are by Yusuf Ali.
18. 2 Kings 6:24–30.
19. For a vivid interpretation of this event and Géricault's painting, see Barnes 1990.
20. Kass 1999:109.
21. Kass 1999:109–10.
22. Kass 1999:110, 112.
23. Much literature exists now on the theology and anthropology of the Eucharist. Two recent examples are Méndez-Montoya 2012 and Wirzba 2011.
24. Dositheus (1672) 2017: chapter 6, decree XVII. Emphasis added.
25. Kass 1999:98.
26. Darwin 1872:256–57.
27. See, for example, Kelly 2011; Curtis 2013.
28. Curtis 2013:3–4.
29. Hygience Centre 2012.
30. John 6:56, and elsewhere.

## 5. EATING

1. Kass 1999:20.
2. Probyn 2000.
3. Jonas 1966:78.
4. Probyn 2000:17.
5. Douglas 2003:30.
6. Levinas 1990:132.
7. Ibid.
8. Plato, *Timaeus*, 70d–71a. For another Platonic version of the tripartite soul, see *Republic*, IX:588c–e.
9. Aristotle, *Nichomachean Ethics*, 3.11.
10. Aristotle, *Nichomachean Ethics*, 10.5.
11. Spinoza 1994:160; see also 175.
12. Plato, *Euthyphro*, 10a.
13. The literature is massive. Some examples are Trayhurn and Bing 2006; Woods 2003; Saper et al. 2002. See also the many studies discussed in Avena 2015; Blundell and Bellisle 2013.
14. Bernard 1974:84.
15. Brillat-Savarin 1999:57. Later he says, "Appetite, hunger, and thirst warn us that our bodies need restorative help" (200).
16. Cannon 1966:59.
17. Chaudhri et al. 2006:1187.
18. Chaudhri et al. 2008:S287.
19. Chaudhri et al. 2008:S287.
20. Dr. Black created this device sometime before 1881, according to the notes of the *Transactions of the Illinois State Dental Society* (Illinois State Dental Society 1895:181). See also *Scientific American* 1911:493.
21. Brillat-Savarin 1999:57.
22. Pavlov 1904.
23. Simpson and Bloom 2010:735.
24. See also Trayhurn and Bing 2006.
25. Brillat-Savarin 1999:57.
26. Brillat-Savarin 1999:182.
27. Cannon 1966:292–93.
28. Peciña and Berridge 2015:125.
29. Peciña and Berridge 2015:131.
30. See discussion by Saper et al. 2002; Peciña and Berridge 2015:134.
31. Conason 2015:156.
32. Kass 1999:115.
33. See discussion of hedonic reactions in Moskowitz 1983:299ff.
34. Brillat-Savarin 1999:200.

35. Jonas 1966:75.
36. Bahya 2010, Second Gate.
37. Plato 1994:81–82 (493e–494c).
38. *Avot d'Rabbi Natan*, 28.9.
39. Sanctorius 1720:331, aphorism 40.
40. For biblical references, see 2 Kings 18:27; Ezekiel 4:12; Isaiah 36:12. For a lighthearted treatment of this eating strategy, see Roach 2013. In elephants, see Guy 1977.
41. Probyn 2000:32.
42. Derrida 1991:115.
43. Derrida 1991:114.

## 6. EATING'S GENESIS

1. Breathing, like eating, takes from the world-not-us, absorbs some of it, and expels what is not consumed along with waste. Both breathing and eating are necessary yet imperfect exchanges with the world.

2. This holds true in the Qur'an, too. Early in *al-Baqarah* ("The Cow"), the second chapter in the scripture, we read, "O ye people! Adore your Guardian Lord, Who created you and those who came before you, that ye may become righteous, Who has made the earth your couch and the heavens your canopy; and sent down rain from the heavens; and brought forth therewith fruits for your sustenance; then set not up rivals unto Allah when ye know (the truth)" (Qur'an 2:21–22). In short, insofar as only God provides for both spiritual and physical prosperity, people should dare not erect false gods.

3. For a classic summary of this model of biblical studies, see Friedman 1987. Freidman (2003) visually demonstrates the Bible's stratified layers.

4. One justification for including the Noahide chronicles as a third creation story comes from a rabbinic opinion fairly widely held. Ravi Abahu taught, "Every time it is written in scripture 'and these' (*va'eleh*), it incorporates what came before, and in every instance when it is written in scripture 'these' (*'eleh*), it disqualifies what came before." One of the versions of the Noah story begins with "these are the generations of Noah" (*'eleh toldot noah*) (Genesis 6:9), meaning that earlier generations—indeed earlier creation stories—are not to be presumed or incorporated. See *Exodus Rabbah* 30.3; *Genesis Rabbah* 12.3.

5. Genesis 1:22. Biblical translations follow the New JPS translation.

6. Genesis 1:26–27.

7. Genesis 1:29–30.

8. For a medieval example of this position, see Bahya ben Asher ibn Halawa, *Shulḥan Shel Arba*, Second Gate, p. 13.

9. Genesis 2:1–4a.

10. Genesis 2:7.

11. Genesis 2:9.

12. Genesis 2:16–17.

13. At the beginning of this section, the text clearly describes this *naḥash* as shrewd ('*arum*), playing on the word for "nakedness" ('*arumim*), which the two human beings embrace unashamedly (Genesis 2:25–3:1). Perhaps the *naḥash* is just as unclothed as the humans. Note, too, in the following verses the *naḥash* is able to speak with the humans (specifically with the woman), and, even more astonishingly, has insights into what God told Adam. Such qualities, abilities, and intelligence suggest that the *naḥash* is more like the humans than not, and that they share a special relation. Even Martin Luther in *Divine Discourses* (§132, p. 64) once described this creature as lofty and noble.

    There is also an orthographic reason to reconsider the nature of the *naḥash*. In the original Hebrew of Torah scrolls, there are no periods indicating where sentences begin or end. Nor are there consistent and clear demarcations of chapter breaks; these were added by the Masoretes in the sixth to ninth centuries CE. Concerning this story, no visible break exists between what we know today as chapter 2 and chapter 3 in the Hebrew text; the next sizable break only appears after Genesis 3:21. This strongly suggests that the famous interaction between the *naḥash* and the woman is part of the same narrative describing the onset of humankind on earth in that special garden. The *naḥash*, too, was there and apparently was perturbed enough to shrewdly get the woman into trouble.

14. There is only one other nonhuman animal that speaks in the biblical corpus: the she-donkey of the prophet Balaam (Numbers 22). For an analysis of that text, see Crane and Gross 2015.

15. Genesis 3:1–7.

16. Genesis 3:9–13.

17. Genesis 3:19. The seventeenth-century English poet John Milton expands upon the fact that what now confounds Adam is eating itself:

    > On *Adam* last thus judgement he pronounc'd.
    > Because thou hast heark'nd to the voice of thy Wife,
    > And *eaten* of the Tree concerning which
    > I charg'd thee, saying: Thou shalt not *eate* thereof, [200]
    > Curs'd is the ground for thy sake, thou in sorrow
    > Shalt *eate* thereof all the days of thy Life;
    > Thorns also and Thistles it shall bring thee forth
    > Unbid, and thou shalt *eate* th' Herb of th' Field,
    > In the sweat of thy Face shalt thou *eat* Bread, [205]
    > Till thou return unto the ground, for thou
    > Out of the ground wast taken, know thy Birth,
    > For dust thou art, and shalt to dust returne.
    > (*Paradise Lost*, 10:197–208)

18. Genesis 3:22–24.

19. And it's messy, when looked at with a fine-toothed philological comb. In Genesis 7:1–5, it is *Adonai*, not *Elohim*, who instructs Noah to bring seven, not two, pairs of each

species and who differentiates clean from unclean animals, a distinction not made in Genesis 6:17–21. The length of the flood is also disputed. In one version it lasts 40 days (Genesis 7:4, 12), while it persists for 150 days in the other (Genesis 7:24). Postdiluvial details similarly differ. Noah sacrifices to *Adonai* pure animals and birds, and *Adonai* quietly articulates a commitment never to destroy the Earth because of humanity's folly (Genesis 8:20–22). The more familiar text has *Elohim* blessing Noah (Genesis 9:1–7). For more on these interlocking authorial voices, see Friedman 1987, 2003.

20. Genesis 6:6–7.
21. Genesis 6:21.
22. Genesis 8:17.
23. Genesis 9:1–7.
24. That this prohibition is reiterated multiple times in the biblical corpus suggests that the desire to consume animal blood was both prevalent and enduring. See, for example, Leviticus 17:11, 14; Deuteronomy 12:23.
25. Genesis 8:20.
26. Genesis 8:21–22.
27. Genesis 9:20–27.
28. The text is curiously silent about what happened on that ark in the first place that inspired God to grant humans permission to eat meat. Though we will never know what that cause was, we do have the subsequent rules about the practice. For one modern meditation on what happened upon the ark, see Barnes 1990.
29. Genesis 6:21.
30. Exodus 16:18.
31. Joshua 1:10–11.

## 7. SATISFACTION

1. Aristotle, *Nicomachean Ethics*, 1127a–1127b.
2. Aristotle, *Nicomachean Ethics*, 1107b4–8; Aristotle, *Eudemian Ethics*, 1230b–1231a.
3. Aristotle, *Nicomachean Ethics*, 1118a.
4. On these peculiar appetites, see discussion in Young 1988.
5. Aristotle, *Nicomachean Ethics*, 1119a16–20.
6. Kant 1996a:267n131. This is found in a paragraph scratched out in the manuscript edition of this slim volume and thus is only infrequently found in published and translated editions.
7. Pitte 1999.
8. For an overview of these kinds of studies of satiety, see Chapelot 2013.
9. See, for example, Rodriguez et al. 2013.
10. Bellisle and Blundell 2013:8.
11. See Smith 1998.
12. Pavlov 1904.

13. Douglas 1972:61.
14. Douglas 1972:67, 69.
15. Douglas 1972:67.
16. Siegel 1957.
17. Levitsky 2013:380.

## 8. JUST RIGHT

1. See Ober 1981 to observe how this story evolved.
2. Deuteronomy 8:17.
3. Deuteronomy 8:18–20.
4. Bahya 2010: Second Gate, p. 5.
5. Deuteronomy 8:3.
6. Deuteronomy 8:10.
7. Deuteronomy 8:12.
8. Bahya 2010: Second Gate, p. 7.
9. These verses are the foundation for the Jewish practice of saying thanks to God after a meal, a prayer known as the *Birkat Hamazon*.
10. 2 Kings 2:11.
11. BT, *Gittin* 70a. This is referenced by the medieval French commentators, Tosafot, BT, *Niddah* 24b, s.v. *achilato merubah mishetayato*.
12. Rashi, BT, *Gittin* 70a, s.v., *achul shalish*.
13. BT, *Gittin* 70a.
14. Rashi, BT, *Gittin* 70a, s.b., *ulchashteka'os*.
15. Maimonides 1964:17.
16. Mishneh Torah (hereafter MT), *De'ot* 5.1.
17. Ibn Ezra on Proverbs 13:25.
18. Proverbs 13:25.
19. MT, *De'ot* 4.1.
20. MT, *De'ot* 4.2.
21. Narrated by al-Tirmidhi, 2380; Ibn Māja, *Aṭ'ima*, 3349; classed as *saheeh* (authentic) by Al-Albaani, in *Saheeh al-Tirmidhi*, 1939; quoted in Al-Ghazālī 2000:6.
22. Al-Ghazālī 1995:127.
23. Al-Ghazālī 1995:108, 110.
24. John 6:11–13.
25. Debate continues about the parallels among Jesus, Elisha, and Elijah. See, for example, Brodie 1981; Evans 1987; Poirier 2009.
26. 2 Kings 4:42–44.
27. BT, *Gittin* 70a.
28. Maimonides 1964:16.
29. MacLean et al. 2015.

30. Pederson et al. 2015.
31. Mattison et al. 2017. See also Martin et al. 2016.
32. Rashi, Leviticus 26:5, s.v., *va'achaltem laḥm-chem lasav'a.*
33. Maimonides 1964:18. See also MT, *De'ot* 4.1 and 5.2.
34. Al-Ghazālī 1995:126–27.
35. Al-Ghazālī 1995:127–28.
36. Medvec et al. 1995.

## 9. SAVORING

1. Derrida 1991:115.
2. Milton, *Paradise Lost*, 9:1017–1021.
3. Milton, *Paradise Lost*, 9:687–690.
4. Serres 2008:154.
5. See, for example, This 2006.
6. Rouquier et al. 2000.
7. Wrangham 2009.
8. Curiously, medieval European art depicts cooking as a collective effort—except in Germany, where for several centuries it was common to show only a single person preparing foods. See "Food Related Paintings," Medieval Cookery, http://www.medi evalcookery.com/paintings.html?germany.
9. Jones 2007.
10. Genesis Rabbah, *Vayera*, 56.3. See also Bahya 2010, Second Gate.
11. Bronowski 1973:125.
12. Though the bonobo Kanzi makes and lights a fire to cook and consume a marshmallow, he was taught by humans to do all this. It remains unclear whether he prefers all, most, or some of his food cooked. "Bonobo Builds a Fire and Toasts Marshmallows," *Monkey Planet*, BBC One, March 26, 2014, https://www.youtube.com/watch ?v=GQcN7lHSD5Y. See also Frontier Gap 2015.
13. This is called the encephalization quotient. See Marino 2013.
14. See Crane 2015; Palagi, Dall'Olio, Demuru, and Stanyon 2014; Rowlands 2012.
15. Serres is not the first to imagine humans with two mouths. Rabbi Shimon bar Yohai in second-century Palestine said, "'If I had been at Mount Sinai when the Torah was given to Israel, I would have asked God to create mankind with two mouths, one to talk of the Torah and one to use for all his needs.' He reconsidered [his suggestion] and said, 'But the world can hardly survive because of the slander [spoken by each person's] one [mouth]. It would be far worse if there were two [mouths for each person]." Jerusalem Talmud (hereafter JT), *Berachot*, 1.2/3b.
16. Serres 2008:153–54.
17. Brillat-Savarin 1999:39.
18. Kant 1996a:§20, p. 44.
19. Brillat-Savarin 1999:40.

20. Upanishads II:2. See Clooney 2011; Seshadri 2011.
21. It is attributed to Avicenna by Benedictus de Nursia in his 1475 *Opus ad sanitatis conservationem*. Cited in Albala 2002:172.
22. Pollan 2013.
23. See Kurlansky 2002; Batterson and Boddie 1972.
24. Probyn 2000:26.
25. Korsmeyer 1999:41.
26. A strikingly similar bowl appears in Brueghels's own pair of paintings on the five senses, *The Senses of Hearing, Touch and Taste* (1618).
27. McFadden 2014:40.
28. Perullo (2016) similarly recognizes that taste is unique to each person. He also promotes the plausibility that taste can be exercised, or trained, through conscientious effort.
29. Barnes 2011:188.


## 10. SACRIFICING

1. Genesis 3:6.
2. Job's comment, "In [God's] hand is every living soul and the breath of all mankind. Truly, the ear tests arguments as the palate tastes foods" (12:10–11), reinforces this theo-ontology of humankind and the centrality taste plays in our very being.
3. Genesis 8:20–22.
4. BT, *Yoma* 83b. This extreme hunger is called *bulmos* in Hebrew, etymologically related to *bulimia*, itself derived from the Greek words *bous* (ox) and *limos* (hunger).
5. 1 Samuel 14:24–30.
6. 1 Samuel 14:27.
7. Rationing for wartime is a common biblical theme. As we saw in chapter 6, Joshua instructs the Israelites to gather rations in preparation for their invasion of Canaan (Joshua 1:10–11). Peacetime rationing also has biblical roots (e.g., Exodus 16:11–18).
8. Proverbs 25:16, 27, 27:7.
9. Muhammad 1967.
10. Exodus 3:8, and many other places.
11. Revelation 10:8–10.
12. Numbers 28, and elsewhere.
13. Genesis 8:21.
14. Psalms 19:10, 119:103.
15. A third possible way to read John's scroll-eating experience is in light of the "Ordeal of the Bitter Water." According to the instructions given in the book of Numbers, a woman suspected of adultery was to be given a watery concoction in which a scroll of curses had been dissolved. If she died because of this bitter water, she was guilty. See Numbers 5:19–23. This unusual trial, if it ever was used, was abolished in the first century CE (M, *Sotah* 9.9). See Grushcow 2005.

16. Genesis 9:20–27.
17. Deuteronomy 32:13–15.
18. For example, Proverbs 23:20; Romans 13:13; Qur'an 2:219, 5:90–91.
19. Ezra 8:10.
20. M, *Avot* 3.17.
21. Qur'an 16:67–69.
22. 1 Timothy 5:23.
23. Qur'an 47:15; see also 76:21, 83:25–27.
24. The blood prohibition arcs back again to Noah. As if giving a concession, God permits Noah and humankind to consume flesh, though only as long as it contains no blood (Genesis 9:4–6). According to Leviticus (7:14), animal blood is to be given over to God and not eaten by humans. The story of King Saul's war against the Philistines (1 Samuel 14:31–35) also speaks about the prohibition of consuming blood. Saul rails against his troops, who sloppily slaughter animals on the ground. He institutes a centralized abattoir and altar to ensure that their herds are appropriately slaughtered and the blood adequately drained. Taken altogether, while animal *blood and fat* are God's, animal *flesh* may be for humans.
25. Leviticus 3:16.
26. Leviticus 7:23–25.
27. Genesis 9:4–6.
28. The book of Leviticus enumerates several kinds of sacrifices. Burnt offerings (described in Leviticus chapter 1) are wholly consumed on the altar; they function for atonement, purification, and thanksgiving. Cereal and grain offerings (chapter 2), also for purification and thanksgiving, require some of the choicest grains to be burned while the rest is given to the priests. Well-being offerings (chapter 3), given for confessions, vows, and free-will gifts, are not to be fully consumed by fire; portions of these sacrifices are to be eaten. Purification offerings (chapter 4) and guilt offerings (chapter 7) are similarly only partially burned and partially consumed.
29. Hill 2011:27.
30. Deuteronomy 31:20.
31. Romans 14:13–15.
32. Romans 14:17–21; compare with 1 Corinthians 10:23–30.
33. Ecclesiastes 1:18; *Ecclesiastes Rabbah* 1.18.1.
34. Bahya 2010, Second Gate, p. 12.
35. BT, *Pesachim* 49b.
36. Bahya 2010, Second Gate.
37. Brumberg-Kraus 1999.
38. Maimonides 1964: chapter 1.
39. *Sunan Ibn Majah* 29.3486.
40. *Sahih al-Bukhari* 5403.
41. See various rates on the USDA's Nutrient Data Laboratory, http://ndb.nal.usda.gov /ndb/search/list.

42. "TRANSforming the Food Supply," *Health Canada*, June 24, 2013, http://www.hc-sc
.gc.ca/fn-an/nutrition/gras-trans-fats/tf-ge/tf-gt_rep-rap-eng.php. See also Ramsden
et al. 2009.

43. This 2006:94–95.

44. Job 6:6.

45. *Sunan Ibn Majah*, 29:3440.

46. Ezra 4:14; Numbers 18:19; Leviticus 2:13; see also 2 Chronicles 13:5.

47. As Kurlansky (2002:7) observes, the Catholic Church dispenses *Sal Sapientia*, the Salt
of Wisdom.

48. Matthew 5:13.

49. Deuteronomy 29:22; Job 39:6; Psalms 107:34; Jeremiah 17:6; Judges 9:45.

50. Luke 14:34–35.

51. Matthew 5:13.

52. Mark 9:49–50.

53. See Leviticus 2:13; Ezekiel 43:24; Ezra 6:9; BT, *Menachot* 20a. In his comment on Leviticus 2:13, Rashi claims that it is because God made a deal with the oceans at the
time of creation that their salt would be used in Israelite sacrifices. (Compare with
Ramban's comment on that same verse.) Salty water, not salty earth, was to fulfill this
vital ritual and sacrificial service.

54. *Bukhari* 7:68.477.

55. BT, *Chullin* 113a.

56. BT, *Berachot* 17b and 34a.

57. Ecclesiasticus 39:25–27 (NRSV).

58. 2 Kings 2:20–22; Ezekial 16:4.

59. JT, *Horayot* 3:6/48.

60. *Sunan Ibn Majah* 16.2567a; compare with Bukhari, *Al-Adha*, 7.68.477.

61. *On Joseph*, §33, §35.

62. BT, *Berachot* 44a.

## 11. SHARING

1. Varro 1912:39.

2. See Robertson et al. 2014:48ff.

3. See Ursell et al. 2012.

4. Ursell et al. 2012.

5. Greshko 2016.

6. Qin et al. 2010.

7. See, for example, Ley et al. 2006.

8. See, for example, Wang et al. 1999; Smith 2015.

9. See, for example, Bravo et al. 2011; Rogers et al. 2016.

10. See Ursell et al. 2012.

11. Goldstein 2013:136.
12. Kass 1999:101.
13. Al-Ghazālī 2000.
14. Matthew 26:17–30; Mark 14:12–26; Luke 22:7–39; compare with John 13:1–17:26.
15. Luke 22:27.
16. Bynum 1987:54.
17. 1 Samuel 1:4–20; BT, *Berachot* 31b.
18. Genesis 18:5.
19. Genesis 43:25, 31; 31:54.
20. Genesis 25:34; 27:17.
21. Genesis 3:19.
22. Levinas 1998a:74.
23. Levinas 1998a:142.
24. Exodus 31:18; Shemot Rabbah 41.3.
25. Levinas 1969:111.
26. Levinas 1969:115.
27. Levinas 1969:114.
28. Levinas 1969:117.
29. Goldstein 2010:37.
30. Levinas 1969:120; Goldstein 2010:37.
31. Online Etymology Dictionary, s.v "Sad," accessed June 29, 2017, http://www.ety
    monline.com/index.php?term=sad.
32. Levinas 1969:33.
33. Goldstein 2010:37.
34. See Goldstein 2010:37; Levinas 1969:118; Levinas 1998a:73.
35. Levinas 1969:117.
36. Levinas 1969:116.
37. Levinas 1969:117, emphasis in original.
38. Kass 1999:41.
39. Levinas 1969:117; see also 129.
40. Levinas 1998a:56.
41. Levinas 1998:74, emphasis added. Derrida (1991) nuances this perspective when he
    says, " 'One must eat well' does not mean above all taking in and grasping in itself,
    but *learning* and *giving* to eat, learning-to-give-the-other-to-eat" (115). For him, eating
    is certainly eating *for* another just as much as it is always an eating *of* an other.
42. Brillat-Savarin 1999:204.
43. Kass 1999:106–7.
44. Julier 2013:3.
45. Goldstein 2013:5. Rabelais (1991) mocks these relations at length.
46. Zohar 3:271b–272a. See Hecker 2000:136.
47. Proverbs 23:1–3.
48. *St. Benedicts Rules for Monasteries*, Rule #53. See Doyle 1948:73–5.
49. BT, *Shabbat* 156b. See discussion in Crane 2011.

50. Midrash Tehillim 119.29.
51. Brillat-Savarin 1999: Meditation 14.
52. Brillat-Savarin 1999: Meditation 14.
53. Serres 2008:163. For more on food sharing, see Jones 2007.

## 12. GO AHEAD, REFRAIN

1. See, for example, Aulus Gellius, *Attic Nights*, edited by John C. Rolfe, §XXIV, Perseus Digital Library, http://www.perseus.tufts.edu/hopper/text?doc=Gel.%202.24&lang=original. Of the many sumptuary laws enacted in ancient Rome, most dealt with expenses related to mealtime consumption. A summary of these rules is available in Harry Thurston Peck, "Sumptuariae Leges," in *Harpers Dictionary of Classical Antiquities* (1898), Perseus Digital Library, http://www.perseus.tufts.edu/hopper/text?doc=Perseus:text:1999.04.0062:entry=sumptuariae-leges-harpers.
2. For example, see Leviticus, chapters 1–5.
3. A Hindi expression, *santripti* or *santrupti,* is often said when one has tasted an incredibly delicious dish or meal. Not based on the quantity one has consumed, it articulates the overarching quality of one's satisfaction. Since the word encapsulates four tastes (sweet, sour, bitter, and salty), it influences the diversity of the 56 (*chhappan bhog*) dishes given as offerings to the deities at New Year's celebrations.
4. Pollan 2011:151.
5. See Swindell 2012, who looked at rats and mice. See also Mattison et al. 2017 in regard to rhesus monkeys; and Longo and Panda 2016, who use animal models to promote age-specific nutrition even in restrictive diets.
6. Martin et al. 2016. See also Parkih et al. 2005.
7. Most et al. 2016.
8. Trepanowski et al. 2017.
9. Fontana and Partridge 2015; Brandhorst et al. 2017.
10. Abassi 2017. Fontana and Partridge (2015) note that genetic differences may also impact a person's response to any diet; no diet proposal—even this one—can or should be assumed to be universally applicable.
11. Pollan 2011:154–55.
12. Ruth 2:14. The Hebrew at the end of the verse, *vatochal vatisb'a vatotar,* means "she ate, she was satisfied, she had left over." The first two verbs link to the verbs of proper satiation Moses champions (Deuteronomy 8:10), as discussed in chapter 8.
13. Ruth 2:18.
14. Goldstein 2013:6.
15. BT, *Baba Metzia* 83b.
16. For a rich discussion on the many ways preventive care outperforms and is more ethically justifiable than reactive care, see Faust and Menzel 2012.
17. Berry 2009.
18. Berry 2009.

# REFERENCES

Abassi, Jennifer. 2017. "Can a Diet That Mimics Fasting Turn Back the Clock?" *Journal of the American Medical Association* (June 28). doi:10.1001/jama.2017.6648.

Adams, Carol J. 2000. *The Sexual Politics of Meat: A Feminist-Vegetarian Critical Theory.* 10th ed. New York: Continuum.

Albala, Ken. 2002. *Eating Right in the Renaissance.* Berkeley: University of California Press.

Ali, 'Abdullah Yusuf. 1989. *The Meaning of the Holy Qur'an.* Beltsville, Md.: Amana.

Allhoff, Fritz and Dave Monroe, eds. 2007. *Food and Philosophy: Eat, Think and Be Merry.* Malden, Mass.: Blackwell.

Aquinas, Thomas. 1947. *Summa Theologica*, parts 1–2. Trans. Fathers of the Dominican Province. New York: Benziger. Dominican House of Studies, Priory of the Immaculate Conception. http://dhspriory.org/thomas/summa/.

Aristotle. 1928. *De Anima.* Electronic Text Center. University of Virginia. http://web.archive.org/web/20080907161558/http://etext.lib.virginia.edu/toc/modeng/public/AriSoul.html. Originally published in The Works of Aristotle Translated into English. Trans. J. A. Smith. London: Oxford University Press.

——. 1934. *Nicomachean Ethics.* Perseus Digital Library. http://www.perseus.tufts.edu/hopper/text?doc=Perseus:text:1999.01.0054. Originally published in *Aristotle in 23 Volumes.* Vol. 19. Trans. H. Rackham. Cambridge, Mass.: Harvard University Press.

——. 1981. *Eudemian Ethics.* Perseus Digital Library. http://www.perseus.tufts.edu/hopper/text?doc=Perseus:text:1999.01.0050. Originally published in *Aristotle in 23 Volumes.* Vol 20. Trans. H. Rackham. Cambridge, Mass.: Harvard University Press.

Aucouturier, J., P. Duché, and B. W. Timmons. 2010. "Metabolic Flexibility and Obesity in Children and Youth." *Obesity Reviews* 12:e44–e53.

Avena, Nicole M., ed. 2015. *Hedonic Eating: How the Pleasure of Food Affects Our Brains and Behavior.* New York: Oxford University Press.

Bahya ben Asher ibn Halawa. 2010. *The Table of Four / Shulḥan Shel Arba.* Trans. Jonathan Brumberg-Kraus. Wheaton College Academic Blogs. http://acadblogs

.wheatoncollege.edu/jbk/shulhan-shel-arba-table-of-contents/translation-of
-shulhan-shel-arba-the-four-legged-table/.

Barnes, Julian. 1990. *A History of the World in 10½ Chapters*. New York: Vintage.

——. 2011. *Pulse*. London: Pace.

Batterson, Mark and William W. Boddie, eds. 1972. *Salt: The Mysterious Necessity*. Pittsburgh: Dow Chemical.

Bellisle, France and John E. Blundell. 2013. "Satiation, Satiety: Concepts and Organization of Behavior." In *Satiation, Satiety and the Control of Food Intake*, ed. John E. Blundell and France Bellisle, 3–11. Oxford: Woodhead.

Bernard, Claude. 1974. *Lectures on the Phenomena of Life Common to Animals and Plants*. Vol. 1. Trans. H. Hoff, R. Guillemin, and L. Guillemin. Springfield, Ill.: Charles C. Thomas.

Berry, Wendell. 2009. "The Pleasures of Eating." Center for Ecoliteracy. http://www .ecoliteracy.org/article/wendell-berry-pleasures-eating. Originally published in *What Are People For?* New York: Farrar, Straus and Giroux, 1990.

Blundell, John E. and France Bellisle, eds. 2013. *Satiation, Satiety and the Control of Food Intake*. Cambridge: Woodhead.

Brandhorst, Sebastian, Eylul Harputlugil, James R. Mitchell, and Valter D. Longo. 2017. "Protective Effects of Short-term Dietary Restriction in Surgical Stress and Chemotherapy." *Ageing Research Reviews*. http://dx.doi.org/10.1016/j.arr.2017.02.001.

Bravo, Javier A., Paul Forsythe, Marianne V. Chew, Emily Escaravage, Hélène M. Savignac, Timothy G. Dinan, John Bienenstock, and John F. Cryan. 2011. "Ingestion of *Lactobacillus* Strain Regulates Emotional Behavior and Central GABA Receptor Expression in a Mouse via the Vagus Nerve." *Proceedings of the National Academy of Sciences of the United States of America* 108, no. 38 (September): 16050–55. doi:10.1073/pnas.1102999108.

Brillat-Savarin, Jean Anthelme. 1999. *The Physiology of Taste: or, Meditations on Transcendental Gastronomy*. Trans. M. F. K. Fisher. New York: Counterpoint.

Brodie, Thomas L. 1981. "Jesus as the New Elisha: Cracking the Code." *Expository Times* 93, no. 2 (November): 39–42.

Bronowski, Jacob. 1973. *The Ascent of Man*. Boston: Little, Brown.

Brumberg-Kraus, Jonathan. 1999. "Meat-Eating and Jewish Identity: Ritualization of the Priestly 'Torah of Beast and Fowl' (Lev 11:46) in Rabbinic Judaism and Medieval Kabbalah." *AJS Review* 24, no. 2:227–62.

Burgand, Deb. 2009. "What Is 'Health at Every Size?'" In *The Fat Studies Reader*, ed. Esther Rothblum and Sondra Solovay, 41–53. New York: New York University Press.

Buzby, Jean C. and Jeffrey Hyman. 2012. "Total and per Capita Value of Food Loss in the United States." *Food Policy* 37, no. 5: 561–70.

Bynum, Caroline Walker. 1987. *Holy Feast and Holy Fast: The Religious Significance of Food to Medieval Women*. Berkeley: University of California Press.

Campbell, Cathy C. 2003. *Stations of the Banquet: Faith Foundations for Food Justice*. Collegeville, Minn.: Liturgical Press.

Cannon, Walter Bradford. 1966. *Wisdom of the Human Body*. Revised and enlarged ed. New York: Norton.

Chapelot, Didier. 2013. "Quantifying Satiation and Satiety." In *Satiation, Satiety and the Control of Food Intake*, ed. John E. Blundell and France Bellisle, 12–39. Oxford: Woodhead.

Chaudhri, Owais, Caroline Small, and Steve Bloom. 2006. "Gastrointestinal Hormones Regulating Appetite." *Philosophical Transactions of the Royal Society Biological Sciences* 361 (June). doi: 10.1098/rstb.2006.1856.

Chaudri, Owais, Katie Wynne, and Stephen R. Bloom. 2008. "Can Gut Hormones Control Appetite and Prevent Obesity?" *Diabetes Care* 31, no. 2 (February): S284–S289.

Clooney, Frank. 2011. "Food, the Guest and the Taittiriya Upanishad: Hospitality in the Hindu Traditions." In *Hosting the Stranger: Between Religions*, ed. Richard Kearney and James Taylor, 139–46. New York: Continuum.

Conason, Alexis. 2015. "The Influence of Dieting (Hedonic Deprivation) on Food Intake, How It Can Promote Hedonic Overeating, and Mindful-Eating Interventions." In *Hedonic Eating*, ed. Nicole M. Avena, 147–61. New York: Oxford University Press.

Crane, Jonathan K. 2011. "Shameful Ambivalences: Dimensions of Rabbinic Shame." *AJS Review* 35, no. 1 (Spring): 61–84.

——. 2013. "The Talmud and Other Diet Books." *New York Times*, March 27. http://www.nytimes.com/2013/03/27/opinion/the-talmud-and-other-diet-books.html.

——, ed. 2015. *Beastly Morality: Animals as Ethical Agents*. New York: Columbia University Press.

Crane, Jonathan K. and Aaron S. Gross. 2015. "Brutal Justice? Animal Litigation and the Question of Counter-Tradition." In *Beastly Morality: Animals as Ethical Agents*, ed. Jonathan K. Crane, 225–47. New York: Columbia University Press.

Curtin, Dean W. and Lisa M. Heldke, eds. 1992. *Cooking, Eating, Thinking: Transformative Philosophies of Food*. Bloomington: Indiana University Press.

Curtis, Valerie. 2013. *Don't Look, Don't Touch, Don't Eat: The Science Behind Revulsion*. Chicago: University of Chicago Press.

Darwin, Charles. 1872. *The Expression of the Emotions in Man and Animals*. New York: D. Appleton.

Derrida, Jacques. 1991. "'Eating Well,' or the Calculation of the Subject: An Interview with Jacques Derrida." In *Who Comes after the Subject*, ed. Eduardo Cadava, Peter Connor, and Jean-Luc Nancy, 96–119. New York: Routledge.

Descartes, René. (1637) 2006. A *Discourse on the Method*. Oxford: Oxford University Press.

——. (1644) 1983. *Principles of Philosophy*. Trans. V. R. Miller and R. P. Miller. Boston: Reidel.

de Solier, Isabelle. 2013. *Food and the Self: Consumption, Production and Material Culture*. London: Bloomsbury.

Donnelly, S. 2008. "Hans Jonas and Ernst Mayr: On Organic Life and Human Responsibility." In *The Legacy of Hans Jonas: Judaism and the Philosophy of Life*, ed. H. Tirosh-Samuelson and C. Wiese, 261–86. Leidin: Brill.

Dositheus. (1672) 2017. *The Confession of Dositheus*. Trans. J. N. W. B. Roberston. Christian Resource Institute. http://www.crivoice.org/creeddositheus.html. Originally published in *Acts and Decrees of the Synod of Jerusalem*. London: Thomas Baker, 1899.

Douglas, Mary. 1972. "Deciphering a Meal." *Dædalus* 101, no. 1: 61–81.

——. 2003. *Food in the Social Order: Studies of Food and Festivities in Three American Communities*. London: Routledge.

Doyle, Leonard J., trans. 1948. *St. Benedict's Rule for Monasteries*. Collegeville, Minn.: Liturgical Press.

Evans, Craig A. 1987. "Luke's Use of the Elijah/Elisha Narratives and the Ethic of Election." *Journal of Biblical Literature* 106, no. 1 (March): 75–83.

Faust, Halley S. and Paul T. Menzel, eds. 2012. *Prevention vs. Treatment: What's the Right Balance?* New York: Oxford University Press.

Fiddes, Nick. 1991. *Meat: A Natural Symbol*. London: Routledge.

Flegal, K. M., B. I. Graubard, D. F. Williamson, and M. H. Gail. 2005. "Excess Deaths Associated with Underweight, Overweight, and Obesity." *Journal of the American Medical Association* 293, no. 15: 1861–67.

Foer, Jonathan Safran. 2009. *Eating Animals*. New York: Back Bay Books.

Fontana, Luigi and Linda Partridge. 2015. "Promoting Health and Longevity Through Diet: From Model Organisms to Humans." *Cell* 161 (March 26): 106–18. http://dx.doi.org/10.1016/j.cell.2015.02.020.

Forth, Christopher E. and Ana Carden-Coyne, eds. 2005. *Cultures of the Abdomen: Diet, Digestion, and Fat in the Modern World*. New York: Palgrave Macmillan.

Freedman, David H. 2011. "How to Fix the Obesity Crisis." *Scientific American* (February): 40–47.

Friedman, Richard Elliot. 1987. *Who Wrote the Bible?* San Francisco: HarperSanFrancisco.

——. 2003. *The Bible with Sources Revealed*. San Francisco: HarperSanFrancisco.

Frontier Gap. 2015. "Animals Who Cook Their Food, and Otherwise Act Very Human." *The Dodo*, February 17. https://www.thedodo.com/animals-acting-suspiciously-li-996022698.html.

Gaon, Sadia. 1948. *The Book of Beliefs and Opinions*. Trans. Samuel Rosenblatt. New Haven, Conn.: Yale University Press.

Gaskins, Ronnesia B., Linda L. LaGasse, Jing Liu, Seetha Shankaran, Barry M. Lester, Henrietta S. Bada, Charles R. Bauer, Abhik Das, Rosemary D. Higgins, and Mary Roberts. 2010. "Small for Gestational Age and Higher Birth Weight Predict Childhood Obesity in Preterm Infants." *American Journal of Perinatology* 27, no. 9: 721–30.

Ghazālī, Abu Ḥāmid Al-. 1995. *On Disciplining the Soul / Kitāb Riyāḍat al-nafs*. Trans. T. J. Winter. Cambridge: Islamic Texts Society.

———. 2000. *On the Manners Relating to Eating / Kitāb ādāb al-akl*. Trans. D. Jonson-Davies. Cambridge: Islamic Texts Society.

Gilman, Sander L. 2008. *Fat: A Cultural History of Obesity*. Malden, Mass.: Polity.

———. 2010. *Obesity: The Biography*. New York: Oxford University Press.

Goldstein, David. 2010. "Emmanuel Levinas and the Ontology of Eating." *Gastronomica* 10, no. 3: 34–44.

———. 2013. *Eating and Ethics in Shakespeare's England*. New York: Cambridge University Press.

Graaf, Cees de, Wendy A. M. Blom, Paul A. M. Smeets, Annette Stafleu, and Henk F. J. Hendriks. 2004. "Biomarkers of Satiation and Satiety." *American Journal of Clinical Nutrition* 79, no. 6 (June): 946–61.

Greshko, Michael. 2016. "How Many Cells Are in the Human Body—And How Many Microbes?" *National Geographic*, January 13. http://news.nationalgeographic.com /2016/01/160111-microbiome-estimate-count-ratio-human-health-science/.

Griffith, R. Marie. 2004. *Born Again Bodies: Flesh and Spirit in American Christianity*. Berkeley: University of California Press.

Grushcow, Lisa. 2005. *Writing the Wayward Wife: Rabbinic Interpretations of Sotah*. Leiden: Brill.

Guy, P. R. 1977. "Coprophagy in the African Elephant (*Loxadonta africana Blumenbach*)." *East African Wildlife Journal* 15, no. 2: 174.

Haslam, David and Fiona Haslam. 2009. *Fat, Gluttony and Sloth: Obesity in Medicine, Art and Literature*. Liverpool, U.K.: Liverpool University Press.

Hatt, J. M. and M. Clauss. 2006. "Feeding Asian and African Elephants in Captivity." *International Zoo Yearbook* 40:88–95.

Hecker, Joel. 2000. "Eating Gestures and the Ritualized Body in Medieval Jewish Mysticism." *History of Religions* 40, no. 2 (November): 125–52.

Heschel, Abraham Joshua. 1993. *God in Search of Man: A Philosophy of Judaism*. New York: Farrar, Straus and Giroux.

Higman, B. W. 2012. *How Food Made History*. Malden, Mass.: Wiley-Blackwell.

Hill, Susan E. 2011. *Eating to Excess: The Meaning of Gluttony and the Fat Body in the Ancient World*. Santa Barbara, Calif.: Praeger.

Hygience Centre. 2012. "The London Disgust Scale." Hygience Central, December. http://www.hygienecentral.org.uk/pdf/London-Disgust-Scale-Dec-2012.pdf.

Illinois State Dental Society. 1895. *Transactions of the Illinois State Dental Society*. Chicago: The Dental Review, H. D. Justi & Son. https://books.google.de/books?id =XRc2AQAAMAAJ.

Irwin, Alec. 2001. "Devoured by God: Cannibalism, Mysticism, and Ethics in Simone Weil." *CrossCurrents* 51, no. 2 (Summer): 257–72. http://www.thefreelibrary.com/D evoured+by+God%3A+Cannibalism,+Mysticism,+and+Ethics+in+Simone+Weil. -a077674977.

Jonas, Hans. 1966. *The Phenomenon of Life: Toward a Philosophical Biology*. New York: Harper & Row.

——. 1984. *The Imperative of Responsibility: In Search of an Ethics for the Technological Age*. Chicago: University of Chicago Press.

——. 1996. *Mortality and Morality*. Evanston, Ill.: Northwestern University Press.

Jones, Martin. 2007. *Feast: Why Humans Share Food*. New York: Oxford University Press.

Jotischky, Andrew. 2011. *A Hermit's Cookbook: Monks, Food and Fasting in the Middle Ages*. New York: Continuum.

Julier, Alice P. 2013. *Eating Together: Food, Friendship, and Inequality*. Urbana: University of Illinois Press.

Jung, L. Shannon. 2004. *Food for Life: The Spirituality and Ethics of Eating*. Minneapolis, Minn.: Fortress Press.

Kant, Immanuel. 1996a. *Anthropology from a Pragmatic Point of View*. Trans. Victor L. Dowdell. Carbondale: Southern Illinois University Press.

——. 1996b. *The Metaphysics of Morals*. Trans. Mary Gregor. New York: Cambridge University Press.

Kass, Leon. 1999. *The Hungry Soul: Eating and the Perfecting of Our Nature*. Chicago: University of Chicago Press.

Kelly, Daniel. 2011. *Yuck! The Nature and Moral Significance of Disgust*. Cambridge, Mass.: MIT Press.

Kemmer, Lisa. 2015. *Eating Earth: Environmental Ethics and Dietary Choice*. New York: Oxford University Press.

Klein, Julie R. 2003. "Nature's Metabolism: On Eating in Derrida, Agamben, and Spinoza." *Research in Phenomenology* 33, no. 1: 186–217.

Korsmeyer, Carolyn. 1999. *Making Sense of Taste: Food and Philosophy*. Ithaca, N.Y.: Cornell University Press.

Kurlansky, Mark. 2002. *Salt: A World History*. New York: Walker.

Leitch, Margaret and Allan Geliebter. 2015. "Overeating and Binge Eating." In *Hedonic Eating: How the Pleasure of Food Affects Our Brains and Behavior*, ed. Nicole M. Avena, 85–105. New York: Oxford University Press.

Levinas, Emmanuel. 1969. *Totality and Infinity: An Essay on Exteriority*. Trans. Alphonso Lingis. Pittsburgh: Duquesne University Press.

——. 1987. *Time and the Other*. Trans. Richard A. Cohen. Pittsburgh: Duquesne University Press.

——. 1990. *Nine Talmudic Readings*. Trans. Annette Aronowicz. Bloomington: Indiana University Press.

——. 1998a. *Otherwise Than Being, or, Beyond Essence*. Trans. Alphonso Lingis. Pittsburgh: Duquesne University Press.

——. 1998b. "Secularization and Hunger." *Graduate Faculty Philosophy Journal* 20, no. 2: 3–12.

——. 2003. *On Escape / De l'évasion*. Trans. Bettina Bergo. Stanford, Calif.: Stanford University Press.

Levitsky, David. 2013. "The Control of Eating: Is There Any Function for Satiation and Satiety?" In *Satiation, Satiety and the Control of Food Intake*, ed. John E. Blundell and France Bellisle, 373–93. Oxford: Woodhead.

Ley, R. E., P. J. Turnbaugh, S. Klein, and J. I. Gordon. 2006. "Microbial Ecology: Human Gut Microbes Associated with Obesity." *Nature* 444:1022–23.

Longo, Valter D. and Satchidananda Panda. 2016. "Fasting, Circadian Rhythms, and Time-Restricted Feeding in Healthy Lifespan." *Cell Metabolism* 23 (June 14): 1048–59. http://dx.doi.org/10.1016/j.cmet.2016.06.001.

Ludwig, Jens, Lisa Sanbonmatsu, Lisa Gennetian, Emma Adam, Greg J. Duncan, Lawrence F. Katz, Ronald C. Kessler, Jeffrey R. Kling, Stacy Tessler Lindau, Robert C. Whitaker, and Thomas W. McDade. 2011. "Neighborhoods, Obesity, and Diabetes—A Randomized Social Experiment." *New England Journal of Medicine* 365:1509–19.

Luther, Martin. N.d. *Divine Discourses*. Trans. William Hazlitt. Grand Rapids, Mich.: Christian Classics Ethereal Library.

MacLean, Paul S., Rena R. Wing, Terry Davidson, Leonard Epstein, Bret Goodpaster, Kevin D. Hall, Barry E. Levin, Michael G. Perri, Barbara J. Rolls, Michael Rosenbaum, Alexander J. Rothman, and Donna Ryan. 2015. "NIH Working Group Report: Innovative Research to Improve Maintenance of Weight Loss." *Obesity* 23:7–15.

Maimonides, Moses. 1964. "Regimen of Health / Fī Tadbīr Al-Ṣiḥḥah." Trans. Ariel Bar-Sela, Hebbel E. Hoff, and Elias Faris. *Transactions of the American Philosophical Society* 54, no. 4: 3–49.

Marino, Lori. 2013. "Humans, Dolphins, and Moral Inclusivity." In *The Politics of Species*, ed. Raymond Corbey and Annette Lanjuow, 95–105. New York: Cambridge University Press.

Martin C. K., M. Bhapkar, A. G. Pittas, C. F. Pieper, S. K. Das, D. A. Williamson, T. Scott, L. M. Redman, R. Stein, C. H. Gilhooly, T. Stewart, L. Robinson, and S. B. Roberts. 2016. "Effect of Calorie Restriction on Mood, Quality of Life, Sleep, and Sexual Function in Healthy Nonobese Adults: The CALERIE 2 Randomized Clinical Trial." *Journal of the American Medical Association—Internal Medicine* 176, no. 6: 743–52. doi:10.1001/jamainternmed.2016.1189.

Mattison, Julie A., Ricki J. Colman, T. Mark Beasley, David B. Allison, Joseph W. Kemnitz, George S. Roth, Donald K. Ingram, Richard Weindruch, Rafael de Cabo, and Rozalyn M. Anderson. 2017. "Caloric Restriction Improves Health and Survival of Rhesus Monkeys." *Nature Communications* 8, no.14063. doi: 10.1038/ncomms14063.

McFadden, Elizabeth. 2014. "Food, Alchemy, and Transformation in Jan Brueghel's *The Allegory of Taste*." *Rutgers Art Review* 30:36–56.

Medvec, Victoria H., Scott F. Madey, and Thomas Gilovic. 1995. "When Less Is More: Counterfactual Thinking and Satisfaction among Olympic Medalists." *Journal of Personality and Social Psychology* 49, no. 4 (October): 603–10.

Melville, Peter. 2004. "A 'Friendship of Taste': The Aesthetics of Eating Well in Kant's *Anthropology from a Pragmatic Point of View*." In *Cultures of Taste / Theories of Appetite: Eating Romanticism*, ed. Timothy Morton, 203–16. New York: Palgrave Macmillan.

Méndez-Montoya, Angel F. 2012. *The Theology of Food: Eating and the Eucharist*. Malden, Mass.: Wiley-Blackwell.

Miller, William Ian. 1997. "Gluttony." *Representations* 60 (Autumn): 92–112.

Mitchell, Stephen. 1992. *The Book of Job*. New York: HarperPerennial.

Morton, Timothy, ed. 2004. *Cultures of Taste / Theories of Appetite: Eating Romanticism*. New York: Palgrave Macmillan.

Moskowitz, Howard R. 1983. *Product Testing and Sensory Evaluation of Foods: Marketing and R&D Approaches*. Westport, Conn.: Food & Nutrition Press.

Moss, Michael. 2013. *Salt, Sugar, Fat: How the Food Giants Hooked Us*. New York: Random House.

Most, Jasper, Valeria Tosti, Leanne M. Redman, and Luigi Fontana. 2016. "Calorie Restriction in Humans: An Update." *Ageing Research News*. http://dx.doi.org/10.1016/j.arr.2016.08.005.

Muhammad, Elijah. 1967. *How to Eat to Live*. Vols. 1 and 2. Phoenix, Ariz.: Secretarius MEMPS.

Murtagh, Lindsey and David S. Ludwig. 2011. "State Intervention in Life-Threatening Childhood Obesity." *Journal of the American Medical Association* 306, no. 2 (July): 206–7.

National Center for Health Statistics. 2012. *Health, United States, 2011: With Special Feature on Socioeconomic Status and Health*. Hyattsville, Md.: National Center for Health Statistics. https://www.cdc.gov/nchs/data/hus/hus11.pdf.

Nietzsche, Friedrich. 2001. *The Gay Science*. Trans. Josefine Nauckhoff. Ed. Bernard Williams. New York: Cambridge University Press.

Ober, Warren U. 1981. *The Story of the Three Bears: The Evolution of an International Classic*. Delmar, N.Y.: Scholars' Facsimile and Reprints.

Palagi, E., S. Dall'Olio, E. Demuru, and R. Stanyon. 2014. "Exploring the Evolutionary Foundations of Empathy: Consolation in Monkeys." *Evolution and Human Behavior* 35, no. 4: 341–49.

Parikh, Parin, Michael C. McDaniel, M. Dominique Ashen, Joseph I. Miller, Matthew Sorrentino, Vicki Chan, Roger S. Blumenthal, and Laurence S. Sperling. 2005. "Diets and Cardiovascular Disease: An Evidence-Based Assessment." *Journal of the American College of Cardiology* 45, no. 9: 1379–87.

Pavlov, Ivan. 1904. "Physiology of Digestion." Nobel Prize. http://www.nobelprize.org/nobel_prizes/medicine/laureates/1904/pavlov-lecture.html.

Peciña, Susana and Kent Berridge. 2015. "Food 'Liking' and 'Wanting': A Neurobiological Perspective." In *Hedonic Eating: How the Pleasure of Food Affects Our Brains and Behavior*, ed. Nicole M. Avena, 125–46. New York: Oxford University Press.

Pedersen, Lene, Rasmus Olsen, Jens Juul Holst, Steen Bendix Haugaard, and Eva Prescott. 2015. "Weight Loss but Not Exercise Lowers Glucagon Response and Improves Glucagon-Like Peptide-1 to Insulin Ratio in Prediabetic Patients with Coronary Artery Disease; The Randomized Cut-It Trial." *Journal of the American College of Cardiology* 65, no. 10: A1511.

Perullo, Nicola. 2016. *Taste as Experience: The Philosophy and Aesthetics of Food*. New York: Columbia University Press.

Pitte, Jean-Robert. 1999. "The Rise of the Restaurant." In *Food: A Culinary History from Antiquity to the Present*, ed. Jean Louis Flanderin, Massimo Montanari, and Albert Sonnenfeld, 471–80. New York: Columbia University Press.

Plato. 1925. *Timaeus*. Perseus Digital Library. http://data.perseus.org/citations /urn:cts:greekLit:tlg0059.tlg031.perseus-engl:70e. Originally published in *Plato in Twelve Volumes*. Vol. 9. Trans. W. R. M. Lamb. Cambridge, Mass.: Harvard University Press.

——. 1966. *Phaedo*. Perseus Digital Library. http://data.perseus.org/citations/urn:cts:greek Lit:tlg0059.tlg004.perseus-engl:57a. Originally published in *Plato in Twelve Volumes*. Vol. 1. Trans. Harold North Fowler. Cambridge, Mass.: Harvard University Press.

——. 1994. *Gorgias*. Trans. Robin Waterfield. New York: Oxford University Press.

Poirier, John C. 2009. "Jesus as an Elijianic Figure in Luke 4:16–30." *Catholic Biblical Quarterly* 71, no. 2 (April): 349–63.

Pollan, Michael. 2008. *In Defense of Food*. New York: Penguin.

——. 2011. *Food Rules: An Eater's Manual*. New York: Penguin.

——. 2013. *Cooked: A Natural History of Transformation*. New York: Penguin.

Probyn, Elspeth. 2000. *Carnal Appetites: Foodsexidentities*. London: Routledge.

Qin, J., R. Li, J. Raes, M. Arumugam, K. S. Burgdorf, C. Manichanh, T. Nielsen, N. Pons, F. Levenez, T. Yamada, D. R. Mende, J. Li, J. Xu, S. Li, D. Li, J. Cao, B. Wang, H. Liang, H. Zheng, Y. Xie, J. Tap, P. Lepage, M. Bertalan, J.-M. Batto, T. Hansen, D. Le Paslier, A. Linneberg, H. B. Nielsen, E. Pelletier, P. Renault, T. Sicheritz-Ponten, K. Turner, H. Zhu, C. Yu, S. Li, M. Jian, Y. Zhou, Y. Li, X. Zhang, S. Li, N. Qin, H. Yang, J. Wang, S. Brunak, J. Dore, F. Guarner, K. Kristiansen, O. Pedersen, J. Parkhill, J. Weissenbach, P. Bork, S. D. Ehrlich, and J. Wang. 2010. "A Human Gut Microbial Gene Catalogue Established by Metagenomic Sequencing." *Nature* 464:59–65. doi:10.1038/nature08821.

Rabelais, François. 1991. *The Complete Works of François Rabelais*. Trans. Donald M. Frame. Berkeley: University of California Press.

Ramsden, Christopher E., Keturah Faurot, Pedro Carrera-Bastos, Loren Cordain, Michel De Lorgeril, and Laurence S. Sperling. 2009. "Dietary Fat Quality and Coronary Heart Disease Prevention: A Unified Theory Based on Evolutionary, Historical, Global, and Modern Perspectives." *Current Treatment Options in Cardiovascular Medicine* 11:289–301.

Roach, Mary. 2013. *Gulp: Adventures on the Alimentary Canal*. New York: Norton.

Robertson, Lesley, Jantien Backer, Claud Biemans, Joop van Doorn, Klaas Krab, and Willem Reijnders. 2014. *Antoni van Leeuwenhoek: Master of the Miniscule*. Leiden: Brill.

Rodriguez, Amia, Victoria Catalán, and Gema Frühbeck. 2013. "Metabolism and Satiety." In *Satiation, Satiety and the Control of Food Intake*, ed. John E. Blundell and France Bellisle, 75–111. Oxford: Woodhead.

Rogers, G. B., D. J. Keating, R. L. Young, M.-L. Wong, J. Licinio, and S. Wesselingh. 2016. "From Gut Dysbiosis to Altered Brain Function and Mental Illness: Mechanisms and Pathways." *Molecular Psychiatry* 21:738–48. doi:10.1038/mp.2016.50.

Romero-Corral, Abel, Victor M. Montori, Virend K. Somers, Josef Korinek, Randal J. Thomas, Thomas G. Allison, Farouk Mookadam, and Francisco Lopez-Jimenez. 2006. "Association of Bodyweight with Total Mortality and with Cardiovascular Events in Coronary Artery Disease: A Systematic Review of Cohort Studies." *Lancet* 368.9536: 666–78.

Rosenblum, Jordan D. 2010. *Food and Identity in Early Rabbinic Judaism*. New York: Cambridge University Press.

——. 2016. *The Jewish Dietary Laws in the Ancient World*. New York: Cambridge University Press.

Rouquier, Sylvie, Antoine Blancher, and Dominique Giorgi. 2000. "The Olfactory Receptor Gene Repertoire in Primates and Mouse: Evidence for Reduction of the Functional Fraction in Primates." *Proceedings of the National Academy of Sciences of the United States of America* 97, no. 6 (March): 2870–74.

Rowlands, Mark. 2012. *Can Animals Be Moral?* New York: Oxford University Press.

Sanctorius. 1720. *Medicina Statica: Being the Aphorisms of Sanctorius*. Trans. John Quincy. London: W. & J Newton. *Google*. https://books.google.com/books?id =eXEFAAAAQAAJ.

Saper, Clifford B., Thomas C. Chou, and Joel K. Elmquist. 2002. "The Need to Feed: Homeostatic and Hedonic Control of Eating." *Neuron* 36:199–211.

Schwartz, M. A. and O. P. Wiggins. 2010. "Psychosomatic Medicine and the Philosophy of Life." *Philosophy Ethics and Humanities in Medicine* 5:2. doi: 10.1186 /1747-5341-5-2.

Schwartz, Michael W., Stephen C. Woods, Daniel Porte Jr., Randy J. Seeley, and Denis G. Baskin. 2000. "Central Nervous System Control of Food Intake." *Nature* 404 (April): 661–71.

Schwartz, Robert M. 2012. *Holy Eating: The Spiritual Secret to Eternal Weight Loss*. Bloomington, Ind.: iUniverse.

*Scientific American*. 1911. "The Power of the Human Jaw: The Work We Do in Biting and Chewing." 105, no. 23 (December 2): 493. https://books.google.com/books?id =KV8IAQAAMAAJ.

Scodel, Harvey. 2003. "An Interview with Professor Hans Jonas." *Social Research: An International Quarterly* 70, no. 2 (Summer): 339–68.

Serres, Michael. 2008. *The Five Senses: A Philosophy of Mingled Bodies (I)*. Trans. Margaret Sankey and Peter Cowley. London: Continuum.

Seshadri, Kalpana. 2011. "Departures: Hospitality as Mediation." In *Hosting the Stranger: Between Religions*, ed. Richard Kearney and James Taylor, 45–54. New York: Continuum.

Shapin, Seven. 1998. "The Philosopher and the Chicken: On the Dietetics of Disembodied Knowledge." In *Science Incarnate: Historical Embodiments of Natural Knowledge*, ed. Chistropher Lawrence and Steven Shapin, 21–50. Chicago: University of Chicago Press.

Shen, Jia, Kobina A. Wilmot, Nima Ghasemzadeh, Daniel L. Molloy, Gregory Burkman, Girum Mekonnen, Carolina M. Gongora, Arshed A. Quyyumi, and Laurence S. Sperling. 2015. "Mediterranean Dietary Patterns and Cardiovascular Health." *Annual Review of Nutrition* 35:11.1–11.25.

Shepherd, Gordon M. 2012. *Neurogastronomy: How the Brain Creates Flavor and Why It Matters.* New York: Columbia University Press.

Siegel, Paul S. 1957. "The Completion Compulsion in Human Eating." *Psychological Reports* 3:15–16.

Simpson, Katherine A. and Stephen R. Bloom. 2010. "Appetite and Hedonism: Gut Hormones and the Brain." *Endocrinology and Metabolism Clinics* 39:729–43.

Sinopoulou, Vassiliki, Joanne Harrold, Jason Halford, and Emma Boyland. 2008. "Meaning and Assessment of Satiety in Childhood." *ECOG.* http://ebook.ecog-obesity.eu /chapter-nutrition-food-choices-eating-behavior/meaning-and-assessment-of-satiety -in-childhood/.

Smith, Andrew F. 2009. *Eating History: 30 Turning Points in the Making of American Cuisine.* New York: Columbia University Press.

Smith, Gerard P., ed. 1998. *Satiation: From Gut to Brain.* New York: Oxford University Press.

Smith, Gerard P, and Graham J. Dockray. 2006. "Introduction to the Review on Appetite." *Philosophical Transactions of the Royal Society, Biological Sciences* 361 (July). doi:10.1098/rstb.2006.1848.

Smith, Peter A. 2015. "Can the Bacteria in Your Gut Explain Your Mood?" *New York Times,* June 23. http://nyti.ms/1N45wIF.

Spinoza, Baruch. 1994. *The Ethics.* In *A Spinoza Reader: The Ethics and Other Works,* ed. and trans. E. Curley, 85–265. Princeton, N.J.: Princeton University Press.

Stuckey, Barb. 2012. *Taste What You're Missing: The Passionate Eater's Guide to Why Good Food Tastes Good.* New York: Free Press.

Sweeney, Kevin. 2007. "Can a Soup Be Beautiful? The Rise of Gastronomy and the Aesthetics of Food." In *Food and Philosophy: Eat, Think and Be Merry,* ed. Fritz Allhoff and Dave Monroe, 117–32. Malden, Mass.: Blackwell.

Swift, Jonathan. 1729. *A Modest Proposal: For Preventing the Children of Poor People in Ireland from Being A Burden to Their Parents or Country, and For Making Them Beneficial to The Public.* Art Bin. http://art-bin.com/art/omodest.html.

——. 1766. *The Journal to Stella.* Ed. George A. Aitken. London: Methuen. https:// www.gutenberg.org/files/4208/4208-h/4208-h.htm.

Swindell, William R. 2012. "Dietary Restriction in Rats and Mice: A Meta-Analysis and Review of the Evidence for Genotype-Dependent Effects on Lifespan." *Ageing Research Reviews* 11:254–70.

This, Hervé. 2006. *Molecular Gastronomy: Exploring the Science of Flavor.* New York: Columbia University Press.

Thompson, Paul B. 2015. *From Field to Fork: Food Ethics for Everyone.* New York: Oxford University Press.

Trayhurn, Paul and Chen Bing. 2006. "Appetite and Energy Balance Signals from Adipocytes." *Philosophical Transactions of the Royal Society Biological Sciences* 361 (June). doi:10.1098/rstb.2006.1859.

Trepanowski, J. F., C. M. Kroeger, A. Barnosky, M. C. Klempel, S. Bhutani, K. K. Hoddy, K. Gabel, S. Freels, J. Rigdon, J. Rood, E. Ravussin, and K. A. Varady. 2017. "Effect of Alternate-Day Fasting on Weight Loss, Weight Maintenance, and Cardioprotection Among Metabolically Healthy Obese Adults: A Randomized Clinical Trial." *Journal of the American Medical Association Internal Medicine* 177, no. 7: 930–38. doi:10.1001/jamainternmed.2017.0936.

Ursell, L. K., J. L. Metcalf, L. W. Parfrey, and R. Knight. 2012. "Defining the Human Microbiome." *NutritionReviews*70(Suppl.1):S38–S44.doi:10.1111/j.1753-4887.2012.00493.x.

Varro, Marcus Terenti. 1912. *Rerum Rusticarum Libri III*. Trans. Lloyd Storr-Best. London: G. Bells. Internet Archive. https://archive.org/details/onfarmingmterent00varruoft.

Visser, Margaret. 1992. *The Rituals of Dinner*. New York: Penguin.

Walker, Michelle B. 2002. "Eating Ethically: Emmanuel Levinas and Simone Weil." *American Catholic Philosophical Quarterly* 76, no. 2: 295–320.

Wang, H., I. S. Lee, C. Braun, and P. Enck. 1999. "Effect of Probiotics on Central Nervous System Functions in Animals and Humans—A Systematic Review." *Journal of Neurogastroenterology and Motility* 22, no. 4: 589–605. http://dx.doi.org/10.5056/jnm16018.

Webb, Stephen B. 2001. *Good Eating*. Grand Rapids, Mich.: Brazos Press.

Wirzba, Norman. 2011. *Food and Faith: A Theology of Eating*. New York: Cambridge University Press.

Wohlleben, Peter. 2016. *The Hidden Life of Trees: What They Feel, How They Communicate—Discoveries from a Secret World*. Vancouver: Greystone Books.

Woods, Stephen C. 2003. "Gastrointestinal Satiety Signals I: An Overview of Gastrointestinal Signals That Influence Food Intake." *American Journal of Physiology: Gastrointestinal and Liver Physiology* 286, no. 1 (December): G7–G13. doi:10.1152/ajpgi.00448.2003.

Woolf, Virginia. (1929). 1989. *A Room of One's Own*. New York: Harcourt Brace.

Wrangham, Richard W. 2009. *Catching Fire: How Cooking Made Us Human*. New York: Basic Books.

Wright, Clifford A. 1999. *A Mediterranean Feast: The Story of the Birth of the Celebrated Cuisines of the Mediterranean, from the Merchants of Venice to the Barbary Corsairs*. New York: William Morrow.

Young, Charles M. 1988. "Aristotle on Temperance." *Philosophical Review* 97, no. 4 (October): 521–42.

Zamore, Mary L., ed. 2011. *The Sacred Table: Creating a Jewish Food Ethic*. New York: Central Conference of American Rabbis Press.

Zeller, Benjamin E., Marie W. Dallam, Reid L. Neilson, and Nora L. Rubel, eds. 2014. *Religion, Food, and Eating in North America*. New York: Columbia University Press.

# INDEX